—THE—
HEALTH
EXPERIMENT

My Intermittent Fasting Story

Finding Sustained Weight Loss,
Health and Peace When Surrounded
by Chaos and Change.

CHERYL GREMBAN

The Health Experiment:
My Intermittent Fasting Story

Cheryl Gremban

ISBN: 978-0-578-81531-2

gremban@sbcglobal.net

This book is dedicated to my family, who loved me regardless of my size and supported every single one of my weight-loss efforts.

TABLE OF CONTENTS

INTRODUCTION

As I sat across from my husband on a date night at a favorite restaurant, he proudly proclaimed, "I am under 200 pounds!"

I smiled at him and acknowledged that I was proud of him, then said, "I am, too." He laughed out loud, not knowing that I, too, weighed in at over 200 pounds not long ago. That was a high point—ugly and brief.

I have lost significant weight several times in my life, but each time I reached a goal—weight or size—the switch was flipped. My eating behaviors changed immediately, and the weight gain began. Just saying I had lost weight implied that I needed to find it or replace it. Sometimes I did both.

This time I dropped the weight and have habits I am willing to maintain forever. This is my story of how my health experiment(s) and intermittent fasting finally got me to a healthy weight that I have maintained for over two years. It is also my story of learning to manage stress, dealing with change, and self-discovery. I am telling you some of my deepest, darkest secrets in hopes that it helps <u>you</u> move forward.

—THE—
HEALTH
EXPERIMENT

My Intermittent Fasting Story

PART ONE:
MY HEALTH EXPERIMENT

JANUARY 2017

183.2 pounds

On January 1st, I was starting my annual New Year Diet—this year I would go back to basics and just count calories. Weight Watchers had allowed me to lose and regain weight multiple times. They were not getting my money this year. I had tried counting fat grams, carbohydrate grams, points, fiber, etc., many times in the past—sometimes with temporary, short-lived results. I had purchased hundreds of books and magazines—all proclaiming the magic cure to my weight problem. None produced the sustained results that I deserved. I had purchased powders, supplements, and meal-replacement shakes that didn't produce the desired outcomes either. So...back to basics and counting calories. Calories in versus calories out was the only truth I knew. Nobody else was going to get my hard-earned money for their empty promises.

I was 60 years old at the time and I had a long history of dieting. My diet history began in my junior year of high school when my father, who always wanted the very best for me, commented that I was getting a little "pudgy" and offered to start a walking program with me. I was probably 5'2" or 5'3" and about 125 pounds. At the time I ate three meals per day and usually only fruit for snacks. I had no idea how to "diet." My mother had dieted off and on while I was growing up (although I only remember her as thin), but I remember very little of what she ate aside from these little candies that were supposed to curb her appetite. They were called Ayds and were an appetite suppressant first sold in the 1930s and 40s and became popular in the 60s and 70s.

She would spend a few hours each week using her "belt massager," which was supposed to vibrate the users to better health, mimicking maximum exercise with minimal effort. I am not sure what results Mom received, but when I tried it, it just made me itch.

That first attempt at weight loss probably resulted in little if any bodily changes but set my brain up for years of body dysmorphia and the resulting yo-yo dieting. I began to notice how thin many of my friends were. They didn't seem to be eating differently than I was. In the summer between my junior and senior years of high school, I began skipping lunch after a small breakfast. I also gave up all "junk" food. My version of junk food at the time included processed sweets and processed salty snacks—chips, pretzels, etc. I still allowed myself fast food and bread, foods that later would be banned in my diets. I was a good little dieter. The weight began to come off. I lost about 20 pounds, and the compliments rolled in.

Sometime in late fall, my perfection "broke." It was like a light switch had been turned back on. I ate a handful of mixed nuts at a party. Those nuts exerted power over me that I couldn't fight back against. The next day, I bought a bag of Circus Peanuts and ate the entire bag—and I would have told you that I didn't really like Circus Peanuts. I had discovered how to binge.

Sadly, my diet/binge cycle went on for years. I have lost significant weight multiple times and little bits even more frequently. I have made attempts to lose a few times each year. Sometimes I succeeded. And then, just as a ball bounces and hits the ground, it rises again. I could never sustain the weight loss.

That is how I once reached over 200 pounds—202 to be exact. I managed to lose some weight and never reached that horrific milestone again. However, I was unable to maintain 140 either. I knew that, statistically, the odds were against me. Research has shown that sustained weight loss is rare. In fact, more than half of lost weight is regained within two years, and 80% is regained within five years (Hall and Kahan 2018). And when you regain the weight, it isn't a secret. It is blatantly obvious just by looking at you. And everyone blames YOU for the weight coming back—including you. I had plenty of experience with weight loss, regain, shame, and self-blame. However, I kept playing the diet game and hoped that someday I would be the winner.

I knew that I was living life in two worlds: life as an obese individual and life with a normal BMI. I was a happy person, but I didn't feel comfortable in an overweight body. I was uncomfortable with my appearance and found my limited activity intolerable at higher weights. I wanted to fully embrace life and participate in all activities. I remember hiking with my youngest son. I always took a camera, even pre-smartphone days. When I became fatigued, I pulled out the camera to stop and capture the moment—view, wildflower, bug, etc. I took as long as I needed to get the perfect photo…and REST.

I heard my share of negative comments toward my body many times in the past. Sometimes, it seems like other people believe if a person is overweight, they are deaf. One time, when I was actually at a normal BMI, an acquaintance called me "fat" to my face. Another time, when I was dressed up (and feeling quite beautiful), a stranger called me a "heifer." Those comments stung me to my core. Although I was not deaf, I was mute. I said nothing. What could I say? I like to think I walked away from both instances with my head held high.

I dreaded having people see me overweight, especially when they last saw me as "normal." I thought it would change their perception of me as a person. When a vacation or special event was planned, I usually mentally calculated the weight I could lose by the event, if I started a diet right then. Unfortunately, I rarely started right then.

As it turned out, I didn't make it through that first day in January within my calorie limit, but I afforded myself some grace because I was out of town. I was still on vacation. Vacations are for enjoyment, right? It was a holiday, and I was celebrating. I told myself I was returning home on the 4th and would restart then. When I failed again on the 5th because there were donuts in the break room, I knew that starting a diet in the middle of the week had to be a mistake. I would wait until Monday to make my perfect start.

THE HEALTH EXPERIMENT

I was so excited on that following Sunday night, as I ate my last supper, lunch, and snacks with all of the junk food that I would be depriving myself of for the next several months. I was ready. My food scale had fully charged, brand-new batteries. My pantry and refrigerator were loaded with low-calorie snacks. And once I had finished the bag of potato chips and dip, the final bit of ice cream from the freezer, and that small bag of M&Ms I had purchased for the occasion, my house would be clear of junk food. If I ate it all that day, I wouldn't have it in the house tempting me tomorrow, and my cravings would be satisfied.

My husband watched as I prepped for my latest diet. He was used to the routine. He never complained about my weight, or the restrictions I put on myself (us) to attempt to lose it. When we were dating, I loved to go to a restaurant that served Weight Watchers food. I loved going out to eat while staying within my dietary guidelines. He hated it but didn't admit it to me until we had been married several years. He confessed to always eating again after those dates.

I woke up on the morning of January 9th ready to slay Goliath, or at least the fat monster. I signed into my calorie-counting app. I was on my way to the perfect body—a long road trip that would be so worth the effort when I arrived. Everyone knows that if I ate less calories than I burned, I would lose weight, right? Apparently, everybody but my body.

I was pretty perfect. There were a few days where I ran out of calories after dinner and ate a little more, but the scale wasn't moving in a way that I wanted it to or believed it should.

I looked at my food journal for possible areas I could improve. I started counting steps in hopes of improving the results. I began journaling my thoughts and feelings each day, hoping my words would hold the solution.

I was a nurse. I counseled patients on how to eat to improve their health. I knew all of the rules regarding eating—even though those rules changed often throughout my career. What was I doing wrong?

I began to look at some of my patients who were younger than I but hospitalized. Many were obese. Would that be my fate soon? I was motivated. I recalculated my BMI at 32.4. I was only a "little obese." Not morbidly so. The good news was that I was down from my previous high weight of over 200 pounds, thanks to some of my former diets.

I continued to count calories and limit what I ate through the month of January. On some days, it looked like I was down a pound, but other days my weight was up. I ended the month at the exact weight as where I began. I was a failure, but I didn't understand why. Counting calories had worked for me in the past, but not this time.

I started to believe that my weight was stuck. I needed to give up attempts at weight loss forever. What I weighed, I would weigh. What I looked like would be my looks. Wide waist and double chins were mine. These were no longer judgements but facts. Unchangeable facts. I had to get used to ME! I could wish myself different—I could dream myself different—but I was ME. Fat me!

I gave up my quest to lose weight. I stopped counting calories but tried to choose healthy foods most of the time. I continued to wear my Fitbit but didn't care how many steps I accomplished. I didn't feel too guilty when I succumbed to a cookie or other "sinful" treat. I continued to weigh myself almost daily so I wasn't surprised to see the scale inch upward.

There was not a specific day that I made the official decision to retire from my life of dieting, but I knew that I definitely had. I no longer binged in anticipation of my next period of food restriction. I quit posting on a social media group that I had belonged to since 2004 in my Weight Watchers days. I wore stretchy clothes so they could grow with me. I didn't succumb to just wearing black, though. I loved bright, colorful clothes and so I wore them.

Yes, I had accepted that I was going to be overweight forever. I figured that I had a big enough personality to go with my obese body. I tried to ignore the nagging thoughts of what negative effects my weight would have on my health. As a nurse, I had vowed to remain on the outside of those hospital bed rails and knew that excessive weight was not helping the cause, but I pulled the curtains of denial.

I knew that I got short of breath walking up hills. My carpal tunnel was causing me increasing numbness and pain bilaterally. I was unable to put on my underwear without leaning against furniture or sitting down. I couldn't balance on one leg. Clothes didn't fit from one season to the next, so I usually only had one piece of each casual clothing. My closet was stuffed full of clothes in so many sizes, but very few of them fit. I was down to a single bra that "fit" and I use that term loosely because, although it fastened, my boob fat hung out in all directions. I had giant front boobs, medium-sized side boobs, and pretty big back boobs. I washed that bra every night and let it dry while I slept. Although I emotionally accepted that I would be fat forever, I was not living my best life. And I avoided both mirrors and photos.

I worked hard to accept this failure point in my life. I was not one accustomed to failure. Usually, I set goals and I met them. What made me so weak that I could not maintain a weight loss?

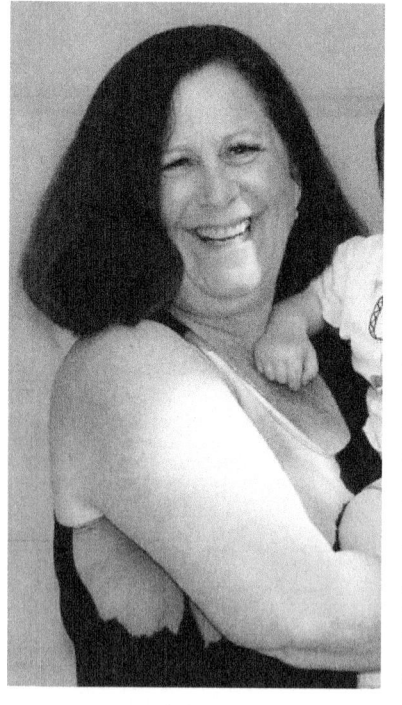

Was it genetic, biological, or was this some personal inadequacy that I had not been able to conquer? I tried to focus on other positive aspects of my life and to ignore my fatness. Crazily, I continued to weigh myself most days—that number brightly shining from my LED scale each morning. I'll admit, those numbers started my day with disappointment. I'm uncertain what I hoped to see— perhaps a miracle of weight loss without trying; my own lottery win!

I had so many positives in my life. I had a husband who loved me regardless of my weight. I had three successful, grown, and married sons. I loved my daughters in law. I had two delightful grandchildren. I had a great job that supported everything I wanted to do. I was able to travel. With so many positives, why did I care about my weight? Even on my worst days, my life was pretty spectacular. However, my body was less than OK.

JULY 2017

178 pounds

I realized that my mindset would be an integral part of my weight-loss journey. I decided that I needed to set goals unrelated to just the scale. I also knew I needed to ignore the calendar—if it took me multiple years to lose the weight, so be it. I would be patient. I would crawl towards my goal. I would remember that even turtles ultimately got to where they'd been heading. Quick fixes hadn't stuck. Perhaps a slow fix would. I had to give up the concept of rewards and punishments regarding food. There were no bad foods—consequently, there could be no good foods. I got to eat what my body wanted. This change in mindset also encouraged more positive self-talk. I gave myself credit for fasting. I promised not to beat myself up if I had a shorter fast or longer eating window or ate "junk food."

In addition, I recognized I needed to start with my beliefs. As Gandhi said:

> *"Your beliefs become your thoughts,*
> *Your thoughts become your words,*
> *Your words become your actions,*
> *Your actions become your habits,*
> *Your habits become your values,*
> *Your values become your destiny."*

I had to believe that I could intermittently fast long term and I had to believe that this way of life would work for me.

My daily journals reflected my love of summer and the daily stresses of my job. Hospitals were facing increased reductions in reimbursements, which led to an attempt to reduce costs. Most employees at my hospital were part of a union, so labor costs were fixed. We were challenged to reduce non-labor costs.

My husband used to say to me each day as I left for work, "Save a life today!" As a non-nurse he didn't realize how much more to the job there was than "just" saving a life. There was handholding, listening to fears, answering questions, praying, and simply sitting quietly at the bedside. This all took time. And, as time IS money, we had to find other ways to reduce hospital costs a penny at a time.

My journal also reflected several days of quality food choices. I was craving salads. I wasn't always grazing through my entire eating window. I was taking more stairs.

I documented my "why." I added to my journal a list of why I was experimenting with intermittent fasting and what I hoped to accomplish:

- I wanted to be as healthy as I could for my grandchildren.
- I wanted to be able to walk up that hill in our neighborhood without stopping to catch my breath.
- I wanted to be able to look over my shoulder while driving to switch lanes safely.
- I wanted to be able to put on my pants without leaning against the furniture.

- I wanted to be able to drive without the numbness in my hands.
- I didn't want the numbness/pain in my hands to wake me up.
- I didn't want to experience cramps in my feet
- I wanted to improve my lipid profile—especially those climbing triglycerides.
- I wanted to feel free of food-choice self-shame.
- I wanted to feel in control.
- I wanted to tolerate the summer heat.
- I wanted to wear shorts in public.
- I wanted to look better in all clothes.
- I wanted clothes to fit from season to season and year to year.
- I wanted to be able to see my jawline when I looked in the mirror.
- I wanted to see muscle definition in my arms and legs.
- I wanted to feel strong.
- I wanted to feel comfortable being photographed.
- I didn't want to suffer from indigestion any longer.

I was finding that intermittent fasting was working for me. I was not eating nonstop around the clock. I was willing to wait for my manageable goal of 16 hours fasting before engaging in the eat mode. I noted that this fasting was producing weight loss. Then, I recognized that I had a few days in a row of excessive hunger and a bit of weakness before my eating window about three weeks into this experiment. This lasted for four days. As quickly as this hunger and weakness appeared, they both disappeared. Thank goodness! I have since learned that this was probably the point in which my body had become "fat adapted"—able to switch to burning fat and not just glycogen. I had graduated to being metabolically efficient.

I was pleasantly pleased with how intermittent fasting was changing my life. Halfway through July, after 30 days of intermittent fasting, I was down 14.2 pounds—now weighing 174.6. I hadn't done anything different except the fasting part. I was motivated by this success. My 30-day experiment was about to extend to 60 days. Intermittent fasting was providing me increased hope for a new body. I rarely had the poo-urgency issues that had plagued me in the beginning. I began to notice my energy increasing. Some days fasting was fairly easy, but other days I found myself watching the clock.

Although I was thrilled that my weight had dropped fairly significantly that first month, I was disappointed that I hadn't dropped a size. My clothes fit better, absolutely. And clothes in my closet that I had not been able to squeeze into prior to starting intermittent fasting were beginning to fit.

I have since learned that my early success with intermittent fasting does not happen to everyone. Many have to heal internally first. Others have to achieve control within their eating window to make intermittent fasting work for them. Holy cannoli! What does having control within your eating window even mean?

THE HEALTH EXPERIMENT

I knew I would need to discover why I overate sometimes. What foods triggered overeating for me? Were there environmental situations that led me to eat more than I wanted? What were some of things I had been told as a child that may have contributed to this behavior?

One cliché many of us heard growing up was: "There are starving children in Africa." This was proclaimed in an attempt to get us to eat our asparagus or to finish whatever was left on our plates. "Don't waste food," was the admonition. I was now aware that overeating does not help those poor starving children in Africa. I also knew that cleaning my plate was just another way of wasting food. The food was still not available for us tomorrow or those starving today.

This made me think about other misleading comments I had heard throughout my life.

I became curious and began to explore the history of frequent meals and the idea that breakfast was necessary. I grew up hearing that breakfast was the most important meal of the day, but breakfast was not always the same, depending on where it was eaten and who was eating it. Most breakfasts were eaten at our home, where cereal was the king. Each week, Mom would take my brother and me to the grocery store where she would plant us in the cereal aisle while she shopped for the rest of our weekly groceries. We wandered up and down the aisle in search of our box for the week. We grew up with Tony the Tiger Frosted Flakes and Toucan Sam's Fruit Loops. I remember my brother leaning toward Captain Crunch each week, while I tended to go for the more mature Life Cereal.

When I had reached the big 1-0 (ten years old), Pop-Tarts became a big part of breakfast. Who could resist a hot pie in the morning? Not me, but it often followed the bowl of cereal. Around the same time, Tang was added to our breakfasts. Tang was a General Foods Corporation product of sugary powder added to water. If it was good enough for the astronauts, it was perfect for kids going to face the adventures of school for the day.

In contrast, on weekends or vacations, when we spent the night at our grandparents', breakfast was different. At Mom's parents, Nana only drank coffee in the morning, and Papa usually had eggs with a couple strips of bacon. At Dad's parents, breakfast was even simpler. Coffee plus toast, but their toast was brown. This was my earliest experience with wheat bread because I grew up in the Wonder Bread era. Wonder Bread had been around since 1921 and became associated with convenience and health in the 1950s. It was sliced and fortified with vitamins. Although my mother was frugal and bought a generic version, our bread was always white. I loved "Nana's bread," as I called it, and begged Mom to buy some of that. Was that my body speaking to me at a young age?

Later I heard: "Eat breakfast like a king, lunch like a prince, and dinner like a pauper." So, did it matter what was on the breakfast menu? And was my coffee, like Nana's, sufficient for the most important meal of the day? Apparently, the idea of breakfast being the best meal of the day was invented by James Jackson and John

Kellogg in an attempt to sell cereal. Later, bacon joined in on the game to add protein to breakfast. So, these slogans came from the food industry. They were not intended to be the absolute truth that we all lived by. But I grew up as if they were!

I have to admit that these revelations caused more questions and increased confusion. I needed to learn more.

Historically, I knew our hunter-gatherer ancestors fasted due to food scarcity. Sadly, they didn't know when their next feast would occur. They hunted meat and gathered fresh fruit and vegetables. They emphasized plant-based foods.

When farming became prominent, ten thousand years ago, three meals a day became the norm. Although food became more available, the variety was sacrificed. Many societies grew a single crop, such as rice or potatoes. This led to a reduction of both height and health.

For centuries, people began to fast voluntarily for spiritual reasons—usually when food was available to accentuate the sacrifice. People of multiple generations fasted for a variety of reasons.

Since I began to accept that I was not hurting myself by skipping breakfast, I had to explore other food myths I heard along the way. I knew that fat had been blamed for widespread obesity, but other food components had also taken a hit. So many types of food have taken the fall for our unhealthy ways. Here are some examples:

EGGS: The history of eggs is complicated and diverse, but humans have consumed eggs for ages. Eggs were once seen as a perfect package of protein and vitamins. Sadly, they were blamed for the cholesterol crisis in the 1960s. Then, 20 years ago, the blame was shifted from the cholesterol in eggs to the cholesterol our bodies made from saturated fats. The resulting condition: one was at risk for was heart disease. Recent studies have shown no increase in cardiovascular disease related to eggs.

BUTTER: I was a youngster when butter took a hit as a major saturated fat source in our diet, and margarine was proclaimed the super substitute (and it was cheaper). The American Heart Association has said that saturated fats should be avoided due to their negative impact on LDL. Margarine is plant based and was supposedly considered healthier until the trans fats it was made of were declared to be the super enemy. So people switched back to butter. Manufacturers have been phasing out the trans fats over the last five years, again instigating the butter/margarine battles.

FAT: In the late 1960s, cholesterol rapidly became public enemy number one, closely followed by its cousin, FAT. Fat had been declared bad for our hearts in 1950 by Ancel Keys, who clearly articulated the results of his
"Seven Country Study," although the results of other countries he studied were not included. This new emphasis on low fat and low cholesterol brought an influx of new low-fat snacks, cookies, etc. These products had decreased fat but increased sugar. This once-vilified food choice has become the hero in "Keto Land." Even

different types of fat have had their days both under fire and in glory. Saturated fats were once heralded as the unhealthy version of fat and now are being touted as a favorite. Polyunsaturated fats, once proclaimed to be a reasonable choice, are now declared to be unstable and inflammatory to the body.

CARBOHYDRATES: In the 1970s, the federal government recommended a high-carbohydrate diet, stating that 55 – 60 percent of calories should come from carbohydrates. The Lancet PURE study showed that both a high carbohydrate diet and a very low carbohydrate diet were associated with increased mortality (Dehghan et al. 2017). The sweet spot seemed to be around 50 percent of calories consumed from carbohydrates. There needs to be a differentiation between complex and refined carbohydrates, however. Fiber, a component of carbohydrates, has been discovered as an essential component to gut health.

ARTIFICIAL SWEETENERS: I will avoid discussing each one separately, but it is important to note that in general they were once held in high esteem, allowing us to enjoy our sweet foods without paying the caloric price. More recently, studies have shown they cause poor gut microbiome health, resulting in increased insulin resistance.

These are examples of the saying that "lies can travel around the world while the truth is still lacing it's shoes." Apparently, our nutritional scientists have been acting as the marketing arm of our food industry. One must dig deep for the truth.

JUNE 2017
188.8 pounds

I had been working as a nurse for 37 years. I had wanted to be a nurse since first grade. At this point in my career, I was a director of nursing in an acute care hospital. My nursing career included many roles: intensive care nurse, school nurse, Medifast weight loss nurse (and, of course, I did that plan), float pool bedside nurse, charge nurse, and nurse manager. I had loved being a nurse and the many roles I had been privileged to do.

Some had called me a workaholic. I worked long hours and was passionate about that work. I loved my patients, but I was really driven to support my fellow nurses. As a nurse, I was only one person, and my impact was limited. However, if I could lead a team with hearts the size of elephants, we could ensure our patients received the care they deserved, and my nurses could go home fulfilled after every shift.

In this role, my days were long, as I carried 24/7 responsibility. I was never "off duty." I was often too tired to worry about the quality and amount of food that I was eating. I frequently found myself feeding my emotions. I had made no further weight-loss attempts since January and remained resolute in my decision to avoid further dieting/weight-loss attempts.

As a nurse I knew about metabolic syndrome. Metabolic syndrome is a collection of risk factors that increase a person's chances of developing heart disease, stroke, and diabetes. Metabolic Syndrome is diagnosed when a person has three or more of the following:

- A waistline of 40 inches or more for men and 35 inches or more for women
- A blood pressure of 130/85 or higher or is taking blood pressure medications
- A triglyceride level greater than 150 mg/dL
- A fasting blood glucose of greater than 100 mg/dL or is taking glucose lowering medications
- An HDL level less than 40 mg/dL for men or 50 mg/dL for women

My waistline had crept up to over 40 inches (check one). I had been taking blood pressure medications for over 10 years (check two). My triglycerides were approaching 150 mg/dL (not quite check three). Fortunately, my blood glucose was fine, and my HDL was optimal. The treatment for metabolic syndrome is to lose weight, exercise, and implement dietary changes. I had ruled out losing weight. I had little time but was willing to consider exercise. And what the heck dietary changes was I supposed to make? Nobody could agree on the rules.

Discussions regarding nutrition seemed to produce a lot of noise and very little substance. The dietary suggestions changed almost as often as I changed clothes. Experts frequently disagreed. What was a health practitioner or patient to do?

I was not typically a cynical person, but I had become quite (OK, I'll admit, VERY) cynical of the diet industry: those who sold services, products, books, magazines, etc., with the promise to lose weight. They sold hope, but the results never materialized for long. If weight was lost, it was soon regained.

In an analysis of multiple weight-loss studies, more than half of the weight was regained within two years and 80 percent within five years. Biological and behavioral aspects conspire to first slow, then stall weight loss. Then the regain begins. The metabolism slows when food is restricted. And behavioral changes return to their original settings as the restrictions persist.

I was not looking for a new diet or eating plan, but this is how intermittent fasting found me. I was chatting with a nurse coworker early one morning at work. She shared that she was starting intermittent fasting. I stared at her, unblinking, and I am sure my look was not entirely accepting. I had never heard of this way of eating before and I was convinced it could not be healthy. And so I blurted, "Are you crazy?"

She laughed at me and told me to google Jason Fung and intermittent fasting. I accepted the challenge and actually looked up the subject right then. I noted there were multiple YouTube videos of significant length so I decided they would need to wait until after work. The day was busy, and I didn't give Jason and intermittent fasting another thought until I was commuting home. I recalled her words: "Jason Fung," "intermittent fasting." What did "intermittent fasting" mean?

A quick rerun of the google search when I returned home yielded the same YouTube videos by the dear Doctor Fung I had seen that morning. Fung is a nephrologist from Canada. As a nephrologist, he was treating those with end-stage kidney disease on dialysis. He recognized that dialysis was just a treatment, not a cure, and began looking for ways he could intervene in his patients' lives sooner. He knew that the leading cause of kidney failure was type 2 diabetes and that obesity was the primary source of that condition. He began his quest to reverse type 2 diabetes and reduce obesity in his patients.

While my husband watched TV, I plugged in my earphones and watched Dr. Fung explain how I could change my life. I loved how Fung expunged me from all guilt regarding my failure to maintain my previous weight losses. He clearly articulated that the calories in versus calories out approach did not work and actually produced many overweight physicians. He forgave me for my failures and blamed the medical community for preaching the same useless lesson for years that did not work. Could I forgive myself? And why, as a health practitioner, had I not been taught the proper way to advise patients—or to help myself?

Jason (I felt like we were on a first name basis at this point) went on to explain that my obesity was a result of excessive insulin. Apparently, as I ate, I also spiked my insulin levels. The more frequently I ate, the more frequently insulin spikes occurred. Insulin causes our bodies to store fat. Each of those spikes causes more hunger. So, I should not be held responsible for often imbibing in that second dessert helping. It also explained why I often ate until I felt sick. He blamed medical professionals for continuously prescribing the frequent-eating plan. That one got to me. I had instructed my patients to do that exact thing. "Repeat a lie often enough and it becomes the truth." Psychologists refer to this as the "illusion of truth effect."

Jason went on to articulate how intermittent fasting could lower insulin, thus reducing weight by diminishing stored fat and decreasing hunger. The science made sense. How could this make so much sense and nobody had ever talked about it before? Later, I would discover some answers to that question. Although I loved the sounds of the science, I was cautiously optimistic.

Dr. Fung went on to explain that we have two sources of energy while fasting. The first source is our glycogen stored within our liver and skeletal muscle. This is the go-to quick energy that our body prefers to use first. The second is our fat storage. Once our glycogen stores are used up, our body will resort to burning our fat. Well, I definitely had some fat to burn. If we ate frequently, we never depleted our glycogen stores. He cautioned that it could take a while to completely deplete our glycogen and begin burning fat. He spoke of a two- to four-week transition period needed to use up our glycogen stores. He offered up the ketogenic diet as a way to speed up the process, but I didn't want to restrict myself to those foods.

I deeply considered this plan for almost five seconds before I knew I had to try it. I imagined a food plan and way of life that didn't restrict foods. I wanted to once again dream of thinner days. I needed to believe that my thinner, healthier self could be unpeeled. I needed to believe this person could remain stripped of her unneeded fat. I needed to hope.

Hope is defined as both a desire and an expectation that something will happen. I had plenty of desire, but my expectations should have been dampened by my previous diet experiences. However, they were not. A study by Chinese psychologists in 2014 demonstrated that hope protects the brain from anxiety (Yang et al. 2014). My hope had a scientific basis.

So, on June 12, 2017, armed with my new intermittent fasting knowledge, I skipped my breakfast, drank a few cups of black coffee, and began my intermittent fasting journey. I began a scientific study, using myself as the one participant. I measured all the data I could think of. I took a selfie. I took the standard measurements and recorded them. I seriously considered the question, "What would my life be like if I fasted 16 hours each day?"

I journaled most days. They were short journal posts, including my morning naked weight, how I felt, etc. I used journaling to note how I was feeling and, most importantly, to see my thoughts. This allowed me to redirect and reframe those negative thoughts as they appeared. I developed a new mantra: "Don't believe everything you tell yourself."

I decided to continue with some of the healthy practices I had attempted in January. I counted my calories but did not overly restrict them. I avoided ultra-processed foods. I gave up wine for the first 30 days. These were frequent practices I had implemented before but had failed to stick with long enough to lose weight. My one change was implementing intermittent fasting. Thus began my study of one: my health experiment.

I had not always been a black coffee drinker, previously preferring cream. When I first switched to the creamless version, it was the look that bothered me the most. Coffee with cream was beautiful and soft in color, whereas black coffee looked stark. I began drinking coffee out of covered mugs to avoid this ugly morning view. I came to discover the taste to be a brisk wake up in my mouth, no longer the gentle ease of morning. I learned to appreciate black coffee. And with intermittent fasting, black coffee gave me sips of success early each day.

It was a Tuesday. I remember it well, partially because I never started anything on a Tuesday. This "diet/experiment" did not begin with a binge because I was not going to totally eliminate food groups. I set a relatively manageable goal of 16 hours fasting. A manageable goal was not too far removed from what I had been doing. A manageable goal helped assure success. If I had chosen a more challenging goal when I began, it may have resulted in failure.

I figured I could do anything for 30 days. I optimistically hypothesized that I would be able to lose weight by intermittent fasting so I was using my weight as the objective measurement for this 30-day test of change. I recorded my weight daily in my journal.

I didn't consider the experimenter bias in my health experiment. Experimenter bias is where the scientist performing the research influences the results in order to portray a certain outcome. I definitely wanted the predicted outcome, but I accepted that although I may be able to influence results temporarily, I would not be able to do so long term.

I will admit those first couple of days were challenging. My brain and body were calling for food well before I was willing to feed it. My commitment to intermittent fasting got me to my eating window. Within days, it was easier. Having the structure of intermittent fasting was helpful, in itself, from day number one. Those donuts in the break room no longer called to me (at least not too loudly) because it was not time to eat. I actually didn't think a lot about food in the morning because I had committed to this fasting lifestyle. I had waves of hunger, but when they were ignored or distracted, those waves of hunger disappeared.

I will admit that when I ate, the food tasted amazing. Better than ever. That, in itself, was a gift. In my overeating days, I had appreciated the relief of anxiety food had offered, the fulfillment of an emotional need, but I don't really recall actually tasting the food.

I made the decision to not talk about my newfound way of living. First, I didn't want to call attention to my obesity. Maybe (hopefully) it was not as obvious to others as it was to me and my scale. Yes, I managed a life of denial quite well. Second, I had started many diets without any success and I had no proof that this would be different. Third, I had lost and regained weight many times, and my friends, coworkers, and family had been witnesses. Would this be different? Fourth, I did not want to defend fasting to anyone. My knowledge was limited. Maybe it didn't work for everyone. Maybe this would be no better than the articles in magazines that had won me over in the grocery store line.

My husband, who was retired, continued to make my "breakfast" of berries and yogurt that I took to work each morning at 6:00 AM. I ate it around noon for lunch—my "breakfast." Notice the word "breakfast" is actually made up of two words— "break" and "fast." So each time you break your fast, you are eating "breakfast," regardless of the time it is eaten or the food consumed.

On the rare occasion when I had a breakfast meeting and food was served, nobody batted an eye when I only drank coffee. These meetings usually had physicians present (food was always served when physicians were present), and I appreciated not being distracted by the food during these meetings.

I could eat my dinner with my husband. He never noticed my health experiment because I was eating real foods and not weighing and measuring every single bite. This was an eating plan that worked for both of us.

I began to love the fasting. Within two to three weeks, my brain felt clearer in the morning. I was totally loving my berries and yogurt "breakfast" at noon. I was very productive. Work was crazy with changes, but I was able to stay on top of it all. I felt calmer in my skin. I continued to journal on most nights. I weighed myself each morning and was happy (ecstatic is the better word) with the trend.

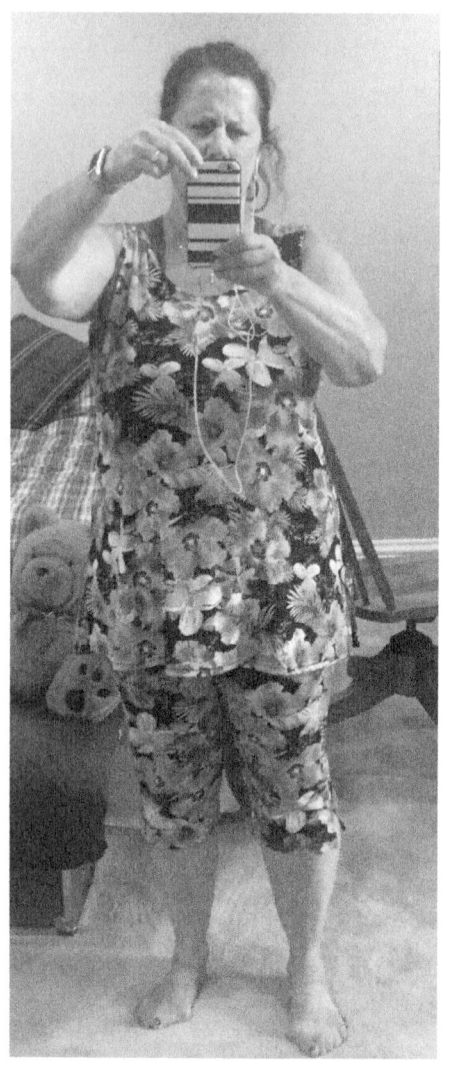

So, here I was, living my experiment of one, secretly, and hoping to revel in its results.

One downside that I noted was a poo urgency within an hour of opening my eating window on some days. Jason hadn't mentioned that in his videos. And my friend hadn't either. Was my body unusual? I have since found out that this is a common side effect of intermittent fasting but of limited duration. But uggggh at the time! I found it best to plan my eating window opening around a time I would be able to use the bathroom. Even with planning, there were times I needed to step out of meetings for that purpose. I accepted this as a side effect of my health experiment and vowed I would work around it.

AUGUST 2017
170.6 pounds

I had lost enough weight that my clothes were looser. My face looked thinner to me, but nobody else had commented on my weight loss. I was finding clothes in my closet that were too small two months ago but fitting now. I was feeling less stress these days—I was not sure why because work was still crazy, but I was calmer. I was no longer bringing yogurt and berries for lunch but regularly buying lunch at the salad bar in the hospital cafeteria. I had enough energy after work to walk the dogs.

I realized I had been experiencing this funky taste in my mouth. It was a combination of lemon and metal. Not at all delightful. What the heck?

Regarding work: Rumors were rampant. Staff's morale was affected. Staff knew that I had always been transparent, but I had no answers. We assumed some announcements were coming, but the persistent silence from leadership was profound. I didn't like how this silence from above was making me look and feel like a director. I wanted to offer more than hugs to my staff. I was unsure that they even believed me when I said that I knew no more than they did.

I have heard it said that our best personality traits can also undo us. I believe my ability to carry out tasks with diligence until their completion was a trait that did not serve me well in the weight-loss game. I diligently worked to lose the weight following the plan of the time. I expected to be "fixed" once the weight was lost and the pounds would magically stay away. I had completed the task at hand with full due diligence. Over and over again, I discovered that it was easier to lose weight than maintain a loss because the pounds always came back.

As Aristotle said, "We are what we repeatedly do. Excellence then, is not an act, but a habit." Intermittent fasting was becoming a habit. A good habit. A great habit that was working for my body. I recognized that we are only a collection of our habits—good and bad.

I could not believe how amazing I felt while fasting on most days. (Some days, though, I was still watching the clock. I was not sure why at the time.) I knew a variety of religions fasted at various times, but I thought that was supposed to be a sacrifice. Was it supposed to feel good? Was it still considered a sacrifice when you felt amazing? How did Nana feel when she skipped breakfast?

Fasting has a long history as a therapeutic regime. The Renaissance doctor Paracelsus referred to fasting as the physician within. Hippocrates, who became known as the father of medicine, believed that fasting enabled the body to heal itself. Now, many years later, I was seeing if that was true for me.

I continued to do internet searches on the benefits of intermittent fasting. I read that in 2016, Yoshinori Ohsumi received the Nobel prize for his discoveries on autophagy. We now know that autophagy is a regulated, orderly process where old broken-down cells are degraded and recycled. Autophagy is stimulated by fasting.

We know that when we eat, insulin increases, and glucagon decreases. Conversely, when we fast, insulin goes down and glucagon goes up to stabilize our blood sugars. It is this increase in glucagon that stimulates the process of autophagy. Fasting also stimulates human growth hormone, which facilitates fat burning as well as muscle gain and an increase of bone density.

Repeated studies have shown that calorie restrictive diets produce adaptive physiological responses that ultimately hinder continued weight release or weight maintenance. Other studies show that intermittent fasting does not produce similar results. So my previous attempts to lose weight had resulted in a slowed metabolism and regain of pounds loss. I was inspired to believe that this time I may be able to maintain the lost weight for longer than 10 minutes.

Intermittent fasting has also been linked to the prevention of multiple diseases: cardiovascular disease, Alzheimer's, some cancers, and type 2 diabetes. Inflammation is also reduced by consistent intermittent fasting. I wondered if my severe carpal tunnel symptoms would be reduced over time with my fasting.

SEPTEMBER 2017
165.6 pounds

When I first began intermittent fasting, I hadn't realized that there were so many different versions and an entire new vocabulary to learn. Intermittent fasting refers to any time periods that result in fasting. In actuality, just fasting during your seven- to eight-hour nightly sleep is considered intermittent fasting. Unfortunately, that fasting length is insufficient to produce the desired benefits of fasting, such as ketosis, clearer brain, energy, longevity, and autophagy.

Time restricted eating (TRE) refers to the time you limit your eating window. That could be anytime from one hour or less to eight hours or more. People typically eat either one meal a day (OMAD) to two meals a day (TMAD) during that time. OMAD typically has an eating window of five hours or less.

Once fasting extends to a second overnight without food, the terminology changes to "no meal days," "up days," "down days," and "alternate day fasting." No meal days can be sporadic or weekly and should be followed by two meals the next day. The rest of the week can have shorter windows. Up days and down days are typically done on a 5:2 plan each week, where two days are either 100 percent fasted or up to 500 calories are consumed. These days are followed by at least two meals the following day.

Alternate daily fasting is simply the 5:2 plan except every other day is a fasting or minimal calorie day.

I was content with my eight-hour eating window. It was working for me. I have since learned that others need shorter windows or up and down days to lose weight. I also developed a strategy that helped me not graze throughout my eating window. Within my eight-hour eating window, I created "windowpanes." These were one-hour periods where I could eat my meals. I started with three windowpanes within my eating window: lunch, a snack, then dinner. I soon learned that I only needed two panes: my lunch of berries and yogurt followed by my dinner.

This was the month I received some unsettling news about work. Our hospital system was facing cost-reduction measures, as were many health systems. This was no surprise to me. I was informed by my boss that I was among a group who would be offered early retirement. I had no clue what that meant—no further details were offered. I have to admit that the news was not totally unexpected, but the lack of details produced anxiety.

My sense of self always had me working until I was at least 65 years old. I had loved working. I had loved my job. The people who I worked with were almost as valuable to me as my family. Was this all at risk?

My husband had finally noticed that I had lost weight. I confessed what I was doing. I expected questions, but none came. He accepted all the eating plans that I tried and this one did not interfere with his way of eating. We could have junk food in the house. We sometimes had pizza for dinner. He often offered me

40

a bite of his snack in the evening and rolled his eyes when I said, "No thanks. My window is closed."

We had a trip planned with some longtime friends to Hawaii this month. I recognized that this would be the first time I would be intermittently fasting outside of my structure of home and work. My mental preparation would be called on to continue successfully on my health journey.

I knew I would have to fess up to them since we were staying in the same condo and they would notice if I was not eating ·breakfast. My friend had recently lost 20 pounds, and she entered the vacation with a no-rule attitude. I entered the vacation with only one rule: I would maintain my 16-hour-per-day fasting schedule. All foods and drinks would be allowed within my window. Nobody was concerned that I did not eat breakfast. I'm not sure they even would have noticed if I didn't tell them. I drank my black coffee as they ate.

I recognized that my structure was not home and work but the actual act of opening and closing my eating window. Sticking with just those acts kept me on track regardless of where I was, the people I was with, or the reason we were celebrating. Life could carry on within that structure. It was magical!

When I returned from vacation, my weight was unchanged. This was a major victory in my book. I had enjoyed multiple foods, lots of wine, and had not gained weight.

Although my husband had noticed my weight loss, nobody else had yet. And although my clothes were feeling bigger and I was able to wear some clothes from the back of my closet, I had not dropped a full size yet—even though my weight had decreased by over 20 pounds. I came to learn that I was probably losing visceral fat—that dangerous fat around my internal organs. I was getting healthier even though my body had not changed as much as I felt it had.

I enjoyed my week away from work, but when I returned, the rumors were still flying. Nobody knew what early retirement meant, and no offers had officially been made. I was handling all of this uncertainty with a relative calmness. Although I had been known for my positivity at work, I usually carried the stress home and unloaded. Not this time. I was able to be positive at work AND at home.

Hormones and proteins have been tied to anxiety and depression. Brain derived neurotrophic factor (BDNF) is a protein found in the brain and periphery noted to be low in depressed patients. Conventional antidepressant medications can raise BDNF. Amazingly, intermittent fasting can increase BDNF by up to 400 percent.

Ghrelin is a hormone that increases when hungry. In multiple studies, ghrelin has been linked to elevated mood. Thus, fasting, and its associated hunger, can result in improved mood. Although many days, I never felt the hunger, there were still some days I did. I celebrated it! I pictured the hunger actually chewing on my fat stores. As I looked in the mirror, I wondered how many meals I had stored in my belly fat, my thighs, my chins.

I was potentially going through one of the most stressful times in my life, as mine was the primary income. My husband had retired several years before, and now my income was in question. Yet I was relaxed and not too worried. I would deal with whatever was to happen.

Many people report increased stress or anxiety at the beginning of their intermittent fasting journeys. I admit that over those first couple weeks, while I was trying to remember to not eat breakfast or steal a donut from the break room, I may have felt some stress. However, once my body adjusted to fat-burning mode and out of glucose-burning mode, fasting became much easier.

I reviewed what Dr. Fung had taught me regarding this magical pathway. I knew that the body could burn both stored fat and glycogen, but that was just part of the story. Apparently, our bodies prefer to burn glycogen because it is easy and quick. This process called glycogenolysis is where the glucagon travels to the liver and converts glycogen back into glucose to be used for energy. This is what my body does each day in the fed state.

The body can only store a limited amount of glycogen—approximately 600 grams. The body will first reach for any ingested glucose first and then reach for the glycogen stores. Once those glycogen stores are depleted, the body MUST resort to fat burning.

Intermittent fasting helps burn through our ingested glucose and established stores of glycogen. Each day, depending upon how long you fast and what is eaten within your eating window, some of that stored glycogen is used for energy, and not all of it is replaced while eating within your window. Within a few weeks, there is no longer enough stored glycogen to get you through the fasting period. That is when the body converts to fat burning.

The benefits are multiple when we finally reach the fat-burning stage. There will be an unbelievable increase in energy and sustained energy. No more mid-day crashes. Mental alertness will peak. Fasting will feel amazing. Apparently, this is where my body was.

OCTOBER 2017
160 pounds

My weight continued to decrease, and I was glad to have something positive to concentrate on because October 2017 was a life-changing month. Within days, I learned that my position was being drastically changed and essentially combined with another position—eliminating one position. All directors were going to have to reapply for their positions—new resumes and day-long panel interviews would be required. Other positions were also being cut within the organization. The early retirement package was not as good as I had hoped. I explored the possibilities of the available positions, even the ones that I knew had been targeted for others. The new position would require that I assume responsibility for two new units and lose responsibility for a unit I had built and was proud of. My career identity was tied to that unit. I knew this change would disrupt the morale on all the units. Nobody liked change. I was uncertain if I was the right person to be the leader of this newly formed team. I admit that I felt vulnerable and uncertain of the direction I should take. There were no sure answers!

I continued to explore all options. I had high expectations of myself in any role. Would I be able to meet my own standards in any of these new positions? Those thoughts kept me awake for a few nights. I considered a conversation with my middle son a few weeks prior when he said, "Mom, you are the most positive person I know, but I have not heard you say anything positive about work in a long time."

When I brought the subject up with my husband at night, he usually would say something like, "You'll figure it out." He didn't attempt to offer advice or lead me to a specific decision.

One evening, I came home from work and said to my husband "What if...I just retire?"

My husband hugged me and said, "I think that is the best idea I have ever heard. Can we move to San Diego?" My husband and I had been considering retiring to San Diego for a couple years, but we didn't expect it to happen for a few years. One of our sons lived in San Diego County with his family. We had a son in New York and one in San Jose as well but could not see ourselves living in either of those cities. I loved the beach. I thought grandchildren would want to visit if they could swim in the ocean, meet Mickey Mouse, and visit LEGOLAND.

The next night, we met with our financial advisor to discuss the feasibility of this decision. We had discussed my retirement in the past, but it had always been theoretical. When we had worked out the actual details, we met with a few realtors to discuss listing our home.

Once we had worked through the logistics, I told my chief nursing officer that I would not be applying for any of the positions and would retire. She told me she understood and we would work out when my last day of work would be—probably mid-December. Part of me wondered why she didn't attempt to talk me out of my decision or change my mind. Was I not the person who should carry on in this new role? Or was she just being supportive of my decision?

When I told my peers (other directors), I received their surprised responses that helped confirm I would be missed. Telling my charge nurses reinforced our mutual appreciation. I needed to believe that I had done well in my role; that I had done the best I could do for my nurses and patients.

My husband and I had been following the available real estate listings in San Diego for a few years. We had limited our ideal retirement oasis to a small area in North San Diego County along the coast. We had recently noticed a listing of a cute 2000-square-foot, one-story home on a small, well-landscaped yard. We decided to drive down on Saturday morning to see the house. The drive took seven hours. We drove directly to the neighborhood and walked around. It felt like home. The next morning, we viewed the house and soon found ourselves in the realtor's office writing an offer to purchase the property. The drive back was seven hours, too, but we were so excited. Our offer was accepted.

I have always known the importance of controlling my stress. Stress produces cortisol. Cortisol is released when the body is perceived to be under stress. Cortisol causes gluconeogenesis, which allows our livers to convert protein to glucose, which results in an insulin spike, increasing our appetites. I was glad these big decisions were behind me and I was ready to move on, but there was so much left to do.

The rest of the month was filled with prepping our current house to sell, negotiating the final details of our home purchase, and telling my coworkers and staff that I would be retiring. I had formed many close bonds. I would miss everyone immensely. The emotions were sometimes overwhelming.

In the midst of this chaotic month, I heard that Dr. Jason Fung had written a book called The Obesity Code. Amazingly, it never dawned on me that there had been a book written about intermittent fasting. I looked it up on Amazon. While looking at that book, I came across several other books written about fasting. Who knew there were actually books written on the subject? One particular book intrigued me. I downloaded a sample of Delay, Don't Deny by Gin Stephens to my Kindle. It was an easy read, so I purchased the Kindle edition. I read the entire book that night.

The book highlighted a version of fasting that Gin now refers to as "clean fasting." To fast clean, one must only consume plain coffee, tea, and water during their fasts. Uh oh! I had been doing it wrong. Although I drank black coffee, I was also sipping low-calorie drinks during my fast on some days. My drink of choice was Crystal Light—fruit punch! Zero calories, but apparently a troublemaker during a fast. Artificial sweeteners could also spike insulin, research had shown (Mathur et al. 2020). I really didn't think it had impeded my weight loss efforts, but I decided to start fasting "clean." I noticed I was no longer hungry before opening my window when I was fasting clean. That is how I "accidentally" extended my fasts to beyond 16 hours.

Gin was a practicer of OMAD—one meal a day, as were many of her followers. I was still happy practicing two small meals per day. I enjoyed a salad at lunchtime with a basic dinner. OMAD was for those people that did not reap the desired benefits from a longer eating window. We all needed to do "our thing." I also noted that I limited my food choices more than others. I saved bread, snacks, and sweets for occasional indulgences. However, I still tended to overeat some sweets if I took that first bite.

Apparently, there is also a Facebook group supporting those who read Delay, Don't Deny and are following the way of life. Could a community practicing intermittent fasting help me in my journey? I loved the idea.

The Facebook group has members who have lost all the weight they wanted to lose as well as many just starting intermittent fasting. I loved seeing the before and after pictures. They were so inspirational. I noted that members ate a variety of foods. I began to wonder if there was a single correct diet and spent time each evening looking for the clues.

I jumped on the "If fasting 16 hours is good, then fasting longer is better" bandwagon. I noticed I was significantly hungrier when I opened my window and ate more quickly. Consequently, I found myself overeating and less satisfied with my food. This part of my health experiment had not worked for me.

On the other hand, if I kept my eating window open for eight hours, I was quite content, even if I only ate for five or six of those hours. Psychologically, knowing I could eat more if my body called for it kept my eating in control during my eating window.

From the books and posts I read, I realized that I am probably unique in my ability to lose weight only fasting 16 hours each day. That said, I was doing what worked best for me.

Halloween came and went. For the first time in my life, or at least since I had teeth, my participation was limited to handing out candy. I did not eat, taste, or sample a single piece. Although my window was open for part of trick or treating, I simply chose to not indulge.

NOVEMBER 2017
158.8 pounds

Some may have been discouraged by the month-to-month weight loss I experienced between October to November, but I recognized the stress (and perhaps overeating) that had occurred in the previous month. I also reminded myself of my commitment to patience on this journey. My house was on the market. I was working to set up my replacement at work for ultimate success. I first thought my successor would come from within the organization but soon learned that those most qualified had chosen not to apply.

I continued to work diligently at my job. It was becoming increasingly apparent that an external search would be required. Those external searches inevitably take a while. I didn't want to leave any loose strings. I owed that to my team. I wanted the best situation for all of them. I offered to participate in telephone screening of external applicants.

In those winter months, I went to work in the dark and came home in the dark. In previous years, the missing sunlight from my workdays produced an internal funk. I began to treat myself to walks outside in the middle of the day. I made up for the time that I walked by going into work earlier or staying later. Those steps in the sunlight brought me contentment and erased any funk that usually enveloped me at that time of year.

I decided to examine the role of the scale in my life. Should I still be weighing daily? Should I believe the results? If I didn't weigh, could I trust how my clothes fit or my measurements? I knew that the scale measured more than just my fat. I knew it included water weight, bone weight, muscle weight, undigested food weight, etc. I considered it a data point. I loved data! I decided to continue to weigh daily and watch the overall trend of the scale. I have since seen the recommendation to weigh daily and average the seven weights for the week to determine a weekly average. Another alternative is to use the app Happy Scale, which does the averaging for you and allows you to visualize future trends (only for iOS users.). When I attended Weight Watchers and weighed weekly at meetings, I would have quit early if that weekly weight was all I had to go by. There were many times when my official weekly weight was up, but on the days before and after my official "weigh in," the scale at home showed lower numbers.

We had a family trip to the Rocky Mountains in Denver the week before Thanksgiving. Since my family is spread across the United States, we like to rent a house in varied locations each year so we can gather as a family. The plan was to celebrate Thanksgiving and hopefully experience some snow. We had both. My husband and I met up with all three sons, their wives, and my two grandchildren (one and a half years old at the time and born 19 days apart). During this trip, my youngest son and his wife announced they would be adding a third grandchild to the mix. While we were in Denver, the grandchildren decided my name would be Mimi. I always thought I would be called Grammy, but the kids had other ideas. Here was another example of life happening despite my plans.

This was my first time with extended family while fasting. I knew what I would say if questions began. Think of our ancestors. They often ate this way. Our body was designed to do this. Do I look healthy? As I made breakfast for the others but did not partake, I was ready for the questions. The only one that came was: "You're not eating?" When I said, "Nope! I no longer eat breakfast," there was no further discussion about it.

I continued to fast "clean." I was back to the 16:8 fasting schedule, no longer experimenting with longer fasts. My kids noted that I looked healthier. I knew the lack of talk about my newest weight-reduction plan was related to the fact that I never retained the loss and I was often experimenting with one plan or another. That said, I was beginning to believe that maintenance of weight loss was possible and perhaps I could intermittently fast forever. I always hoped for that possibility, but uncertainty had persisted.

My house received three offers over list price while we were enjoying family time in Denver. We chose to accept one of them. Life was changing in many ways. We would be moving on to our dream of living near San Diego.

It snowed some while we were on this trip. The grandchildren, who had not experienced snow, were now doing so. They were young and not overly impressed.

This was the month that fasting seemed to be effortless on all days. The lack of sugar-free drinks during my fast had made the difference. Apparently, my body was releasing insulin with those drinks, resulting in increased hunger. I had not correlated my challenging fasts with the days that I was consuming my artificial drink of choice—Crystal Light. No more artificially sweetened drinks in my fast eliminated the need to white knuckle until my window opened.

The funky taste in my mouth was receding. I read that the taste was probably from being in ketosis, so I feared I was losing ketosis as the tastes faded. What I hadn't realized was that as my body became more efficient at burning ketones, the funky tastes abated.

DECEMBER 2017
154.8 pounds

I hadn't been told when my last day of work would be. When I asked my boss, she told me to ask Human Resources. When I asked Human Resources, they said it was up to my boss. The position had not been posted yet to external applicants. Obviously, the expectation was I would work beyond mid-December.

I had a move date for January 8th. I applied for a week vacation and started developing a backup plan in case I was not released from my duties. Since I was accepting a reduction in force, I needed to be let go from my position. I found a room in a local home I could rent, if needed. I would move to Southern California and then return to the Bay Area Monday through Friday until I was "reduced" from my job.

I spent all my free time shopping for online Christmas gifts and purging a lot of things that had accumulated in the 20-plus years we lived in this house. We sold a few items through my work's weekly news. We made frequent trips to Goodwill to donate boxes of unneeded items. Some things we just put out on our driveway with a free sign. Most disappeared quickly.

I was amazed at how much we had accumulated in the 20 years we had been in this house. I found six and a half pairs of snow boots for my husband. That's right. Not only were we holding onto a single errant boot; we held onto six pairs. We lived in an area that did not receive snow. We visited snow only every few years. Crazy!

That said, I had clothes in my closet from size 6 to 16. Maybe even crazier!

I was determined that my new home would be less cluttered and simpler. That said, I held onto the boxes of size 8 clothes that I was committed to wear again. I felt like I was getting close. I actually had very few clothes that fit me well at the time.

I was excited to live a simpler life—less stuff around me. I hoped that this simpler life would flow easily with intermittent fasting. I wanted to feel more alive, surrounded by fewer material items. External clues are powerful. Studies have shown that people eat more when surrounded by clutter than they do in a tidy environment.

Coworkers all noticed my weight loss now, and the questions were coming. How had I lost the weight? What was intermittent fasting? Was I sure I was getting enough to eat? I explained that I had several meals stored on my thighs. I also confessed I was still counting calories.

I knew that counting calories was not a recommended strategy to be used in conjunction with intermittent fasting, but I had been hesitant to give up this crutch. I did note that my counting was not always accurate. I tended to stop counting when I ran out of calories and still wanted to eat. I often underestimated the size of a portion of a desired treat—calling a cup of ice cream a half a cup, for example, when documenting what I was eating. I rarely weighed and measured my food.

What I hadn't realized was that caloric counts were based upon 19th century laboratory experiments and considered flawed by many researchers today (Howell and Kones 2017). Apparently 1,000 calories for me may not be 1,000 calories for you. How much energy does each of our bodies expend to break down a given food? How does our differing gut bacteria aid in our digestion or rob us of some of those calories for their own use? How was the food prepared? Food preparation affects caloric content. Has the food evolved to avoid digestion? Oh my! So many factors to consider. Dr. Fung says, "Calories exist in physics, not in physiology," which is a fancy way of saying calories exist in a science lab but not in our bodies. Our bodies process nutrients, not calories.

All my adult life, I had allowed labels to dictate the value of a food, regardless of the plan I was following. The following study reminded me that labels are not just labels; they evoke specific beliefs. Alia Crum's study on milkshakes offered insight (2011). Crum made a giant batch of vanilla milkshakes, divided them in half, and labeled each half differently. The first half were labeled a low-calorie drink with zero percent fat, no added sugar, and only 140 calories. The second half were labeled as an incredibly rich treat with enough sugar and fat to equal 620 calories. In truth all milkshakes had 300 calories each. She measured the ghrelin before and after the study participants drank their milkshakes. Ghrelin is referred to as the hunger hormone, secreted by the gut, telling a person they are hungry and slowing their metabolisms. Once a large meal is consumed, the ghrelin drops. Scientists have always thought that ghrelin levels fluctuate based upon actual food eaten. Crum found that the levels were dependent upon what the person believed they consumed. She noted the ghrelin dropped three times as much in those who drank the "indulgent" shakes over those who drank "low-calorie" drinks.

If I didn't count calories, how would I know when to stop eating? Those who had done intermittent fasting long term suggested listening to their bodies. I wasn't sure that my body could speak, let alone in a language I understood, but I was willing to try. I figured that this would be the perfect month to add another facet to my health experiment. I would not count calories and tune into what my body was telling me. I set a goal to enjoy some holiday treats and maintain my weight at the same time. If I could do that, then I stood a chance of being able to sustain a weight reduction.

Each morning when I woke up and prepared for the day, I considered what holiday treat I would indulge in that day. It was exciting to have so many options. One day was fudge. Another day was eggnog. Still another day was pasta and garlic bread. Gradually, I began to hear the faint voice of my body telling me when I was satisfied and if the food I had just tasted was worth it.

During this holiday season, I considered all the gifts my body has given me:

- The ability to wake up each morning

- The hands to make coffee and the taste buds to enjoy every single sip
- The fingers to tie my shoes and button my blouse
- The coordination to drive a car
- The feet to walk into work
- The brain to solve problems
- The teeth to chew my chosen foods
- The eyes to see the beauty that surrounds me
- The ears to hear my grandchildren call me "Mimi"

I could go on and on. Although I have not always been thrilled with the shape and size of my body, it has always supported me.

JANUARY 2018
153.4 pounds

This New Year did not involve another resolution to lose weight. Yes, I had more weight to lose, but I was convinced that I would get there doing intermittent fasting. What a relief to not be looking for a new diet this year. What JOY!

When I returned to work after the New Year, I was officially told that my last day of work would be January 5th—I would not need my back up plan. I was going to retire; be reduced.

I was thrilled with the results of my last health experiment. I had not gained weight over Christmas—partaking in the treats with no attempts of calorie counting. Could I finally be free of this task?

I was ready to move on to my next health experiment, and my oldest son had chosen the specific element—-alcohol. We were to all participate in Dry January. I would have no wine this month. Ugggggh! With the pending move, I was unsure that I wanted a wine-free month, but this was my family's way of supporting my weight-loss efforts. On the bright side, I hoped they were correct and this was what my body needed to release some more weight and get closer to goal.

I knew that alcohol could contribute to weight gain or sabotage weight loss efforts. First, alcohol is calorically dense, containing seven calories per gram. (Fat contains nine calories per gram and protein and carbohydrates each contain four calories per gram). Alcohol is more quickly stored as fat than fat, protein, or carbohydrates. Whereas foods can take a long time to digest, alcohol is digested quickly. This rapid digestion of alcohol can produce low blood sugar, which results in us overeating. In addition, alcohol impairs the prefrontal cortex of the brain—that area in the brain involved in decision making—leading to less than favorable food choices.

I completed my last week of work. Reports were written. Rounds were made. Suggestions were given. Who knows how much of that work was deemed important to others, but it was important to me. I knew that I would miss these people. My team was another family to me.

My staff threw me a party upon my exit. We celebrated in a restaurant. I wanted to tell them how I believed that they made me a success, but words failed me. I knew I would never forget them. Sadly, I don't think I adequately conveyed their importance in my life. I continue to hope they just knew...

The actual move to San Diego County went quite well. The pack-up of our house by the moving company was done, amazingly, in one day. I followed the packers and cleaned along the way. At the end of perhaps the longest day in my life, I settled into a hotel room with my dogs, waiting for my husband to bring our fast-food dinner.

The next day, we drove our own separate cars to our new home. The rain poured. I had our girl dog in my car, and Hubby had the boy dog in his. Our first stop was coordinated, but due to the intense rain, we decided to navigate separately the rest of the way. Although we had been close to one another for the first part of the trip, my Google map took me in a different direction than my husband's after the stop. Surprisingly, we showed up at our end destination hotel within 15 minutes of each other. My eating window had been short on that move day because I did not want to stop again for food. And there was no wine when we reached the hotel.

My dogs were unbelievably happy in the hotel. We spent a couple nights there while we waited for our furniture to be delivered to our new home. We had no snack food in the hotel, so my eating was limited to meals out and the free breakfast at the hotel (food unworthy of my window.) My husband would indulge in the Belgian waffles while I sipped my black coffee in the morning. I experimented with a few longer fasts: 18 – 19 hours but ultimately reverted back to my 16:8 schedule. That schedule had been working well for me, and I feared setting myself up for failure by pushing my fasts longer. My brain had been trained with years of diet failures and continued to search around each unknown corner for the next reason to trip up.

Once the moving van arrived at the new home, and we unloaded everything, we were ready to transition to our new life. We met new neighbors. We explored new walking trails. I found the hills very challenging at first but vowed that someday I would hike them with ease.

My body needed sleep. I complied. After years of long hours, I was able to give my body what it wanted—hours of undisturbed sleep.

I had received a Christmas Gift of DNA testing with 23andMe. I sent in my vial of saliva, not knowing what to expect. My profile included significant health information, also. Apparently, according to my DNA report, saturated fats were worse for me that the average person and could cause significantly more weight gain. No wonder those donuts and chips stacked up the pounds on my body. I also was genetically predisposed to age-related macular degeneration but not Alzheimer's, Parkinson's, or type 2 diabetes. My DNA reported that I was likely to weigh less than the average female my height and have the muscle mass of a power athlete. Yeah, sure! Explain that to my remaining fat and lack of muscle. I was still above normal BMI.

FEBRUARY 2018
144.6 pounds

The lack of wine and the reduction of stress combined to produce a fabulous weight release over the last month. Although I didn't miss the stress, I did miss the wine and looked forward to adding a little back into my way of eating.

It was time to start getting realistic about my goal weight. My original goal had been 145. All my size 8 clothes fit me. I felt good about myself. However, I was still at the top of my BMI normal range. I knew I should lose a little more, but I wasn't sure how much more. I wanted a weight that I could easily maintain. I never wanted to be faced with a mountain of weight to lose again.

I decided that 140 would be a more realistic and healthy weight for me. I also believed that my body would know when it had reached its goal by not giving up any more weight. I was going to trust my body.

I really tried to listen to what my body was telling me. I worked to eat until satiety. That was a new one for me. I used to eat until stuffed and more recently ate to full. I was unsure what satiety felt like. I allowed myself to predict my satiety by eating a smaller portion, then waiting. If I was still hungry, I ate a little more. After a while, I became quite adept at predicting the amount of food I needed to satisfy myself.

Some people speak of a "sigh" when their body was satiated. I hadn't heard or felt that yet, but I still seemed to know.

I realized that the new people I was meeting had no idea that I once (or multiple times) was obese and had a history of yo-yo dieting. I didn't introduce myself as "Hi. I'm Cheryl. I used to weigh over 200 pounds. I've lost weight lots of times, but I can't keep it off." I simply went with "I'm Cheryl. We just moved in." If I managed to keep the weight off, these people would only know me as "normal BMI Cheryl."

Hubby and I began the work of relearning how to live together with neither of us escaping to work for long hours at a time. We no longer had the subject of the move or my job to discuss over dinner. We spent time dividing up the household duties. We saw several movies in the theatre (Movie Pass was big at the time), sometimes calling popcorn our dinner. We sometimes went to the gym together, where he did his thing (the elliptical) and I tried to figure out what my thing would be. I tried yoga, Pilates, and Zumba. I liked yoga the best. We talked about places we would like to travel. We debated whether to watch sports or the latest Netflix hit on TV at night. We sat out back and listened to our wind chimes and fountain after dinner, while drinking (wine for me and beer for him) and living the dream. We took turns choosing different restaurants to try for date night. It was so fun to explore our new community in this way without worrying about dietary restrictions.

The next step was to literally step.

The Health Experiment

I lived in an area of coastal beauty surrounded by hills and beautiful hiking trails and nature. I increased my exploration of my new town by walking. I walked in every direction from my house. I had some favorite routes, which I walked frequently. My step count was now well over 10,000 steps every day. I looked forward to my walking tours. I learned to meditate while walking, concentrating on my breaths or tuning into the nature around me. Those steps brought me peace and internal joy.

To walk more than two miles in any direction from my house required ascending a wicked hill. One of my first attempts was a walk to the beach, which was three miles away and required climbing one of those wicked hills. I put Hubby on call, in case I needed a ride home. As I moved up that hill, I took my time. I turned around a couple times, noting the distance I had traveled. I was awestruck. I focused on how far I had come, rather than how far I had to go. I made it to the beach, where again, I was moved by the beauty surrounding me. I texted my husband and told him that I didn't need a ride. I walked back home.

My steps had become as important to me as fasting. I learned to exercise in the fasting state, and it felt incredible. I began my exercise routine with walking because it was easy—it met me at my current fitness level and required only shoes as equipment. It was another manageable goal that I could succeed at.

We have often heard that 10,000 steps per day is the goal to improve health. Here is another area where the goal was driven by marketing, not medicine. In 1965, a Japanese company launched a pedometer with the slogan of (loosely translated) "Let's get 10,000 steps per day." That number had stuck as the default for other fitness trackers. A study of over 16,000 women, undertaken 2011 – 2015 showed that walking just 4,400 steps each day resulted in a 41% reduction in mortality compared to walking just 2,700 steps per day. Walking 7,500 steps each day resulted in a 65% reduction (Lee et al. 2019).

In a separate study published in Journals of the American Medical Association (Saint-Maurice et al. 2020), the above information was confirmed. This study used a sampling of Americans over 40 years of age and showed that taking 8,000 steps per day was associated with a 51% reduction in mortality and taking 12,000 steps each day was associated with a 65% reduction of risk.

Studies have shown that exercise is beneficial for health but won't aid in weight loss if the diet remains unchanged (Cox 2017). I hoped that intermittent fasting combined with my steps would turn out to be the one-two punch I needed to lose a little more weight and maintain that loss. I was off to another health experiment on myself.

So far in my health experiments with a sample size of one (me), I had learned the following:

- Intermittent fasting—following a 16-hour fast and an 8-hour eating window—allowed me to lose weight
- I didn't need to count calories to lose weight
- If I gave up alcohol for a period of time, my weight loss increased
- Stress reduction helped my weight-release efforts

THE HEALTH EXPERIMENT

I wonder what else I could learn about myself during my health experiments.

I noticed that my self-talk affected how I moved about my day. When I spoke negatively to myself, fasting was harder and I ate more in my window. When I gave myself kudos or spoke in a neutral tone, my fasts were easier and food consumption in my window was more reasonable.

I needed to work on my brain to banish some those ingrained diet thoughts. I regularly had to remind myself that food wasn't good or bad. Consequently, I was neither good nor bad based upon foods I had consumed. I knew my mindset would play a part in my weight maintenance. I began to ask myself questions. What did I really want to eat? How would my future self (myself one hour from now) think of the decision I was making now? Would my future self be happy with the decision to eat that chocolate chip cookie? I also began to practice gratitude toward my body. Instead of noting the persistent areas of flab and cellulite, I began to note how easily my body carried me on a three-mile walk, the areas of muscles that were forming around my back and shoulders, and how the many aches and pains that were once present had vanished.

MARCH 2018
141.6 pounds

I was almost under 140 pounds and feeling quite pleased with myself. I was never going to quit intermittent fasting, but I was allowing myself more frequent "treats" these days. I had become much more selective about my treats. I preferred ice cream and potato chips to baked goods.

My body had been pretty talkative lately. I heard it requesting me to vary my vegetables each day—apparently, I shouldn't live on green beans alone. The meal planning had become challenging. My husband and I decided that one of those meal delivery services could work for us. If you haven't tried them before, meal delivery services send you all of the ingredients that you need for each particular meal. We chose the three meals per week plan. We tried two different companies—Blue Apron and Home Chef— before finally settling on Home Chef.

I admit there were times I got a little cocky and experimented with chips, jellybeans, chocolate, etc. One day, as I shopped at Costco, I noticed that the giant container of Jelly Bellys was on sale. Of course, I bought one. I had full intentions of controlling my intake. I started out with a small handful. Then another. No matter how hard I tried, I ate more Jelly Bellys than I had planned for or wanted. I tried moving the container into another cupboard. That did not reduce my consumption. Then I moved the container to the trunk of my car. Unbelievably, I grabbed my car keys several times during my window, went out to the garage, and grabbed another handful of those candies. What was wrong with me? After a few days, I finally threw the remainder away. It was obvious that I could not control my intake of that sugary snack. This was a lesson that I needed my body (and my brain) to remember. I have now come to believe that foods that I can't control well probably spike my insulin, resulting in further hunger for the same food.

One of my favorite tools was journaling. I had been journaling since January 2017, so this entire "experiment" had been documented. I have frequently reread posts to determine what was working versus what was not. It helped me keep track of my goals and progress towards them. It was a place to keep track of measurements, labs, fasting time, photos, etc. Some days I recorded only a sentence or two. Other days included a few paragraphs.

Here was one of my recent posts: *"3/30/18. 139.2 pounds. My weight has not been this low since 2015, and that was short lived. I can feel my hip bones. Wow! Today was a walk day—4 miles on my favorite trail. I also added a yoga class. BP 101/65. Fasted 16.5 hours without difficulty. Tonight I made a new shrimp fajita recipe. Definitely repeatable."*

Journaling helped me discover which foods I couldn't stop eating once I started: candy and cookies, especially. Journaling also helped me discover that eating pizza and pasta can be controlled within my window but make me hungrier the next day. Journaling helped me discover that ice cream can be controlled within my window and does not make me feel hungrier the next day but is not helpful in the weight-loss process. Journaling helped me to discover that eating a mostly whole foods diet serves me best when trying to lose weight.

Journaling also helped me to discover that sugary, ultra-processed foods made me feel sluggish and unmotivated. I accomplished less on days that included these foods on the menu. Amazingly, foods with natural sugar, such as fruit, produced the opposite results—energy and productivity. All this helped me to limit my added sugar intake and use fruit to manage my sweet tooth.

My favorite result from journaling was recognition of negative thoughts as they creeped in and the opportunity to reframe them. Throughout my journey, my negative self-talk came less frequently, but I anticipated a potential surge of negativity as I entered maintenance.

I visited the Bay Area and had the opportunity to stop by my former place of employment. Everyone said that I looked younger and that retirement agreed with me. Many said that they missed me and the place was not the same without me. What went unspoken was that it would not have been the same, even if I had stayed with all the ongoing changes. My former coworkers had survived. My leaving had very little impact on their lives. They continued to use their elephant-sized hearts to provide quality care to their patients.

When I returned home, I began exploring diets related to longevity. There are people who live in five regions of the world known for longevity—many living beyond 100 years old. I wanted longevity as long as it could be combined with relative health. I explored many of their habits. They move their bodies a lot. They participate in communities. They take time and find ways to limit stress. They are committed to their families.

These Blue Zone communities, as they are called, are relatively free of heart disease, cancer, diabetes, and obesity. I considered which of my habits were Blue Zone habits. I moved a lot; I was often getting over 15,000 steps each day. I felt like I belonged to a community and I was committed to my family. I limited the amount I ate.

What were the areas where my habits did not coincide with the Blue Zones? I still indulged in some sugary or salty snacks—a Blue-Zone no-no. I ate meat at most dinners. Was I willing to make any changes in these areas?

I decided my occasional indulgence in a sweet or salty treat, I would maintain. However, my husband and I decided we would be happy eliminating meat from our dinners a couple nights per week and including more seafood.

I began exploring vegetarian recipes. We discovered we loved quinoa, farro, and grits. We found out that many of these recipes took extra preparation time because of all the chopping required. We also learned that our grocery bill went down.

APRIL 2018
138 pounds

I was glad to be under 140 pounds. My weight release had definitely slowed down, but I didn't mind. I was at goal. I had clothes that fit. I packed away all my big clothes for donation. I continued to love intermittent fasting and I was never going to quit. I was ready to practice maintenance, but I was unsure how maintenance compared to what I had been doing the past several months.

I considered the last few times I had binged. They weren't frequent anymore, but there were specific foods that when I thought of them, I couldn't visualize myself just eating a single portion. I knew that if I started eating those foods, I would not stop until they were gone or I felt sick. Donuts, candy, and cookies had been the frequent culprits. What do these foods have in common? Primarily sugar.

Dr. Bert Herring had done extensive work around appetite correction and fasting. He has over 20 years of personal experience and thousands of years of user experience following a 19:5 window. He believes that our appetite centers know when to stop eating. Fasting can activate our once-inactive appetite centers. He also mentions for many people, sugar can temporarily deactivate their ability to recognize satiety. I, apparently, am one of those people.

A funny thing happened after several months of intermittent fasting. I rarely craved sugar or other junk food anymore. My body began to crave healthy foods—foods that were easy to not overeat. And foods that reacted well with my body.

Yoga was a frequent addition to my regular exercise routine. I had never been flexible, so yoga was a challenge for me. I also liked the relaxation elements of it. I still practiced planking on days I didn't do yoga. I planked during commercials of my favorite TV shows.

Was I always perfect? Absolutely not. Some days I ate beyond satiety because I was enjoying the tastes, the feel of the food in my mouth. However, I accepted my humanness and started over from there. Some studies have shown that if a person eats healthy most of the time, the body adjusts to rare short-term periods of overeating by shifting the metabolism to use that excess food. The secret is to assure that these bursts are short and infrequent. Call it a metabolic boost and move on.

I was shopping at our lovely farmer's market one morning, when I inadvertently accepted a sample piece of cheese. Then panic set in. I was supposed to be fasting. It was not time to open my window. I took a few deep breaths, accepted my imperfection, realized I was not hungry, and continued my fast. Intermittent fasting had taught me there was no on/off switch and no wagon to fall from. I could be imperfect. I could have longer eating windows on some days. And I was still intermittent fasting. What a gift!

I realized that willpower was not as big a factor in intermittent fasting as it had been in diets I had attempted throughout the years. In those diets, my willpower was required 24 hours each day to restrict foods and their amounts. With intermittent fasting, when willpower was needed, it was only needed for part of each day and then it could rest while I was in my eating window. Since willpower appears to be limited, the rest period gave my willpower bank a chance to build its reserves. As time went on, willpower was rarely required because my body and brain (conscious and unconscious parts) were on the same page.

I was happy and busy with my new life of retirement, but I struggled to find a sense of purpose. Would volunteer work fill that need, or did I need a part time job? What would keep me busy and content?

MAY 2018

133.8 pounds

How did I get here? The last time I weighed this little, I was training for a marathon in 2004 and counting points with Weight Watchers. Before you begin thinking I am an elite athlete, I need to confess that at that time I had never run over one mile in my life. I was not a runner. I had tried a couple times—that is where the one mile had come from. But one day, I got in my head that I wanted to complete a marathon.

My original goal was to walk 26.2 miles—the actual length of a marathon. As I began researching marathons, I discovered that most had very strict time limits. I was unlikely to make those limits by walking. So then I began intense research for a marathon with longer time restrictions. Thank you, Internet!

I found the Honolulu Marathon had no time limits. Check. I noted there was a training program in my area. Check, check. This particular training program raised money for people suffering from AIDS, and my sister in law had died from AIDS several years before (from a blood transfusion). Check, check, check. I went to an information meeting and signed up.

The day I told my husband that I wanted to run a marathon, he asked me if I knew how far that was. I told him "Yes—26.2

miles." He said, "Maybe we should get in the car and drive that far first."

When I signed up, I knew that I was expected to raise significant money for AIDS. I was uncomfortable asking for money if I was ONLY walking. So, I decided to try to learn to run. We were going to do three miles at our first meeting, which was two and a half months away. I set out to learn how to run three miles. UGGGH!

I discovered a run/walk format promoted by Jeff Galloway, a famous marathon runner. I decided I could learn to run four minutes and walk one minute. Before long, I had worked myself up to three miles and was ready for my first marathon meeting.

I trained hard for several months to work up to marathon distance. In the process, my weight dropped from the upper 130s to the lower 130s. I completed that marathon in December 2004 in just under five and a half hours. Then, just as quickly as I started running, I quit. I was burnt out. And my weight climbed from there.

Now here I was in the low 130s without running. There was nothing to quit except intermittent fasting, and there was no way that was going to happen. I was on a roll. I felt fantastic. Was fasting my superpower?

There was a time when I believed that dieting was my superpower. Give me a diet, and I could follow it. When other people said that they had tried XYZ diet but didn't make it beyond two to three days, I could proudly proclaim that I was well into my second month. What I didn't admit is that, often, the weight loss had already stalled and the regaining had begun.

After I began additional reading on longevity, wellness, and intermittent fasting, I learned that I wanted my superpower to be my ability to delay the onset of chronic diseases. Fasting was just one part of the equation.

I knew from the very beginning of my health experiment that I needed to lose weight to get healthy. I also knew there had to be more to it. It is believed that 25 percent of variation in the human lifespan is determined by genetics. Obviously, there is no way for any of us to impact our genetic pool after we are born.

The other 75 percent is determined by the following lifestyle practices:

- Avoid overeating—intermittent fasting should help in this area.
- Eat some nuts—this is a food I had avoided for years related to its fat content. Nuts are rich in protein, fiber, antioxidants, magnesium, potassium, and multiple vitamins. They have been associated with a longer lifespan.
- Eat plenty of plant foods. This seems to be a no brainer for both fiber and vitamins, as well as antioxidants.
- Stay active—although the type of activity and length and frequency of activity vary by study.
- Don't smoke and moderate alcohol intake seem to be the consensus these days.

- Develop a good sleeping pattern. A recent study reports that longevity is associated with sleeping at least seven hours each night and going to bed and arising around the same time each day (Mazzotti et al. 2014).
- Avoid chronic stress as much as possible.
- Maintain both happiness and social circles.

So, intermittent fasting was only part of the story. We must focus on other areas to reduce disease and live longer.

I began exploring other activities for both fitness and fun. We had pickleball courts in the neighborhood. Hubby and I took a few lessons and had fun chasing that little ball. We also had a pool. I began swimming some laps. Although the hills challenged me, I began riding my bike some. These were fun activities that didn't feel like exercise.

So, I am glad that I started small with my activities and built from there. And now I needed some new clothes. My size 8s were now too big.

JUNE 2018
129.8 pounds

I was below 130 pounds. I don't remember weighing this little for any extended period since high school. I may have briefly weighed this when I got married, but I had dieted to get there and began the regain process on our honeymoon. I decided this was going to be my new goal weight. I was finally at the weight that had been written on my driver's license since I moved to California over 20 years ago. My body knew what it wanted to weigh as I entered that field on my license application. I had just never gotten there.

What made me think that my brain was ever in charge of my goal weight? Does my brain decide how fast I will run a mile? Does my brain decide how big my feet will grow? My body has always had its own decision-making power, and weight goal is part of that power.

I was approaching my one-year anniversary of intermittent fasting. I had only hoped for such changes. I began to seriously consider that I could maintain this weight. I knew I could and would continue intermittent fasting.

The best parts of intermittent fasting were the increased enjoyment of food and the freedom from always thinking about and judging food. In the days prior to intermittent fasting, I was always thinking about and fearing food. What should I eat? How much should I eat? Can I really eat that? Will that make me fat? Those internal discussions were no longer a part of my day. I broke my fast with a small meal (I was back to berries and yogurt on most days) and then I ate dinner a few hours later. I ate to satiety. I allowed foods to nourish me; to satisfy me. I chose foods I liked. Most of those foods I would consider healthy, but I didn't judge. If I wanted pizza, then I ate pizza. If I wanted dessert, I ate it.

I have read a lot about how our gut microbiome affects the amount of energy extracted from the food that we eat. Had my gut microbiome changed? Was I able to eat more than I had before?

I usually still fasted 16 hours per day on most days and had an 8-hour eating window. That continued to work for me. I've heard that it does not always work for others. I think it is because I consistently got a lot of steps in my day and ate primarily foods that were not ultra-processed. I enjoyed fruits, vegetables, meat, fish, nuts, grains, and dairy on a regular basis. My body called for less sugary or salty snacks, but I still indulged on occasion. I also enjoyed having wine.

I was in love with fasting! I considered my fasting schedule as my body's healing time. I began to think there would be days that I fasted longer so that I would have more time to heal. I wanted the healthiest gut possible. I wanted to live a long time and maximize my quality of life. I hoped that autophagy would protect my brain health and tighten some of my loose skin. Some said that autophagy had healed their periodontal (gum) disease. This was an area that would benefit me. I read an article that the polyphenols in coffee induced autophagy. Tea and decaffeinated coffee offered the same benefits. I added some tea to my daily routine.

People have asked me how I avoided eating all day long when I was retired and at home. Just like people who work all day away from home, I made a list of all I wanted to accomplish before I ended my fast. On that list I included my workout, household chores, errands, and social time. This list provided structure to my day and kept me from mindlessly eating.

I began my intermittent fasting life simply and without many tools. I used my Fitbit to count steps and measure my sleep. I still weigh daily. I measure every couple months. I use my camera to see what the scale and measuring tape don't capture. I still journal regularly.

Since I had reached my goal weight, I decided my next challenge would be to find my next purpose in life. I explored a variety of volunteer opportunities. I applied for a few part-time jobs. I began babysitting more.

JUNE 2020
119 pounds

So much has changed in my life! Intermittent fasting has been the one constant. We have completed three months of shelter in place during the COVID-19 pandemic. Although some entities are opening up, life remains far from normal. My gym is closed. My pool is closed. I have been unable to travel—even to visit my out-of-the-area grandchildren. Trips to New York, Northern California, and Africa have been cancelled. I can't even sit on my beautiful beach. Through all this, intermittent fasting has been my calming, settling force.

Many refer to this time as the Pandemic 15 or COVID-15—the weight they gained during this uncertainty. Some have chosen this time to delay their progress, rather than continue or begin their self-work toward health. I have chosen to continue fasting and limit my eating window. My weight now fluctuates between 117 and 122. I was able to maintain my weight with intermittent fasting and steps. Just prior to shelter in place, I renewed my license with a documented weight of 120. On that day, the listed weight was a bit of lie because I weighed 119 that morning.

My weight has never again gone over 130 and has been steady for almost two years. I finally reached the goal my body chose. My BMI was now safely in the normal weight category, although I recently discovered I was only 5'3" instead of the 5'4" I thought I had been.

I have not been sick since beginning intermittent fasting. I have always been relatively healthy and was happy to remain so. I continue to fast daily. I usually aim for 18 hours and sometimes make it to 20. Some days, I acknowledge my humanity and only fast for 16 or 17 hours. I continue to shake it up and keep my body off balance. I have never done a fast of over 24 hours. I continue to utilize the windowpane strategy on some days, if needed.

I am glad my weight is within the normal limits because obesity is a major risk factor related to COVID infection, hospitalization, and death. People who are obese have a 46% greater chance of becoming infected by COVID than those of normal weight. These same obese people have a 113% higher risk of hospitalization, 74% higher risk for ICU admission, and 48% higher risk for death (Popkin et al 2020). Was my weight release protecting me from COVID?

In the picture on the next page, my typical self-care has not occurred. I have not had a cut and color, and my greys are visible. I have not had a manicure or pedicure. However, I still feel beautiful, healthy, and strong.

Many of my size 6 clothes can be removed without unzipping them. I am unsure what my actual size is these days. I have size 4s that fit and size 4s that are too big. I also have size 2s that fit and size 2s that are loose. I just bought my first size 0 and was amazed to see that they fit. Who knew that my body would continue to change so dramatically after my weight was fairly stable?

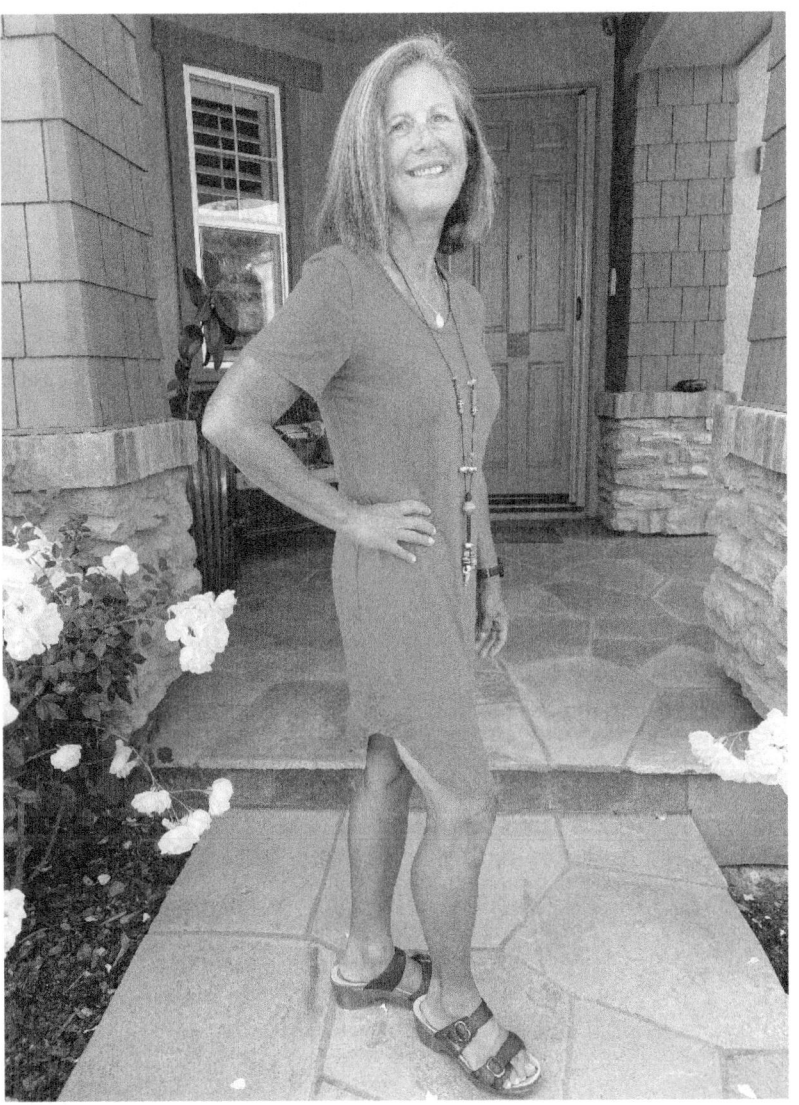

My Birthday 2020 — 64 years old

Regarding what size I actually wear, I have no clue! Women's sizes are crazy! That said, it is sort of fun saying I fit into a size 0. Thank goodness I continue to take measurements and can buy clothes online using the size charts.

I now had five grandchildren, with a sixth on the way. They have been an integral part of my life. Intermittent fasting allows me to be in the best shape to keep up with them. They are active. My former body would have struggled with keeping up, getting off the floor, carrying them. Now, although exhausting, I can manage full days with them.

Although those first videos by Jason Fung on intermittent fasting declared it to be a lifestyle, I was unsure if I actually bought into that at first. I was committing to a 30-day health experiment, which I extended multiple times. Somewhere before the first-year mark, I knew that I had committed for life. There would be no turning back.

This plan is doable. This plan is flexible. This plan meets me on every special occasion, holiday, and vacation, and we make it work. I sometimes have longer eating windows. I sometimes eat ice cream. I sometimes (but rarely) eat nothing considered "healthy" in a given day, but I am still intermittent fasting.

My three-year fastiversary is this month. I still have no desire to stop. I love how I feel when I fast. I love that I have maintained my weight loss for about two years. I am a statistical anomaly as a dieter, but a typical intermittent faster. I no longer feel controlled by food. As Kim Smith (author of Unbelievable Freedom) would say, I have finally found freedom from the grasp of food addiction, extra-large body, and the dieting game.

There have been days when I first wake up and I don't recall those years of being overweight. Believe me, the memories usually come soon after, but I no longer dwell on them or feel ashamed by them. They are a part of me. I feel AMAZING. I don't think I have ever felt better.

I handle what life throws at me and deal with it with strength and grace. That alone (even without weight loss) makes intermittent fasting the best thing I have ever done—my best gift.

I have continued to weigh myself daily and use the Happy Scale app. The log below shows a recent week. Notice the daily weight column versus the moving average. Although my actual weight varies from 117.8 to 121.6, my moving average remains consistent in the 119s and 120s.

	RECORDED	MOVING AVERAGE	LOSS/WEEK
	JUNE 2020		
08 Mon	118.8	119.1	0.8
07 Sun	119.8	119.2	0.7
06 Sat	120.0	119.2	0.8
05 Fri	118.4	119.2	0.7
04 Thu	117.8	119.5	0.6
03 Wed	119.2	119.9	0.3
02 Tue	120.8	120.2	0.2
01 Mon	120.2	120.3	0.1
	MAY 2020		
31 Sun	120.8	120.5	—
30			

I upgraded my scale this last year to one that includes more than just weight. Many proclaim their relative accuracy compared to the expensive DEXA scan. I love seeing multiple numbers, especially that metabolic age. I doubt I will continue to get metabolically younger, but I love being four years younger than my actual age.

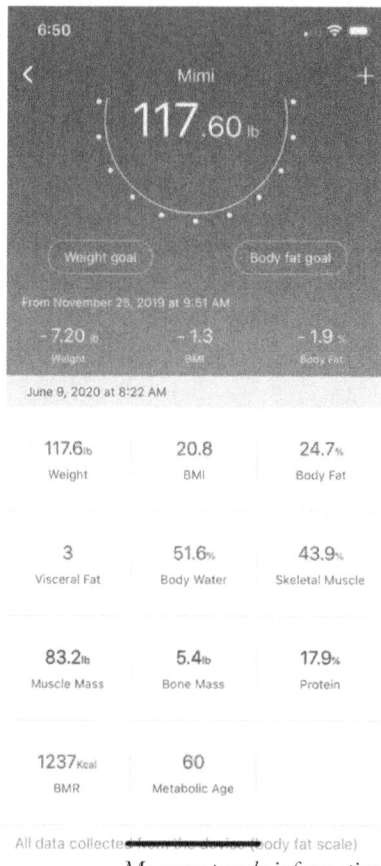

My smart scale information

The Health Experiment

Some people do not weigh at all and use other information, such as measurements or goal pants, to keep them on track. I love the data from my scale and I have fun trying to predict what it will say. I typically lose two pounds overnight. Pizza for dinner will result in a small gain the following morning. I will lose one half pound running fasted.

All this said, scales vary on their accuracy. I remember the scales of my high school days through the early 2000s. I could lean one way to make it go up and another way to make it go down. I could have a scale reading six pounds apart depending on my leaning direction. In 2003, I purchased a new scale that was unswayed by my leaning methods. My scale became more of a truthsayer. My current smart scale also ignores attempts to skew the results.

I mentioned many of my scale victories above. Listed below are my measurements. Although I didn't lose the same number of inches from each area, I made my body look proportional. When I look at photos, I would have thought that I lost the most from my breasts, but actually I lost more from my waist. My 36DDDD bra size, which I would have proclaimed as breast-reduction worthy, has settled into a 32DDD and seems to fit my body.

Before and After

Measurement	Before	After
Bust	44.5"	36"
Waist	40.5"	26.5"
Hips	46"	35.5"
Lt. Thigh	28"	20.5"
Lt. Arm	14.5"	10"

My waist to hip ratio went from 0.88 (high risk for type 2 diabetes, heart disease, and some cancers) to 0.75 (low health risk). Women should be at or below 0.80 to maintain low risk. Men should be at or below 0.95. My waist to height ratio went from .64 (considered highly obese) to .42 (considered slender and healthy). See chart below.

Waist / Height
ratio

0.58 and over	0.63 and over	▶	Highly Obese
0.54 - 0.58	0.58 - 0.63	▷	Extremely Overweight
0.49 - 0.54	0.53 - 0.58	▷	Overweight
0.46 - 0.49	0.46 - 0.53		Healthy
0.42 - 0.46	0.43 - 0.46	▷	Slender & Healthy
0.35 - 0.42	0.35 - 0.43	▶	Extremely Slim
0.35 or below	0.35 or below	▶	Abnormally Slim

The Health Experiment

I was glad I had taken measurements. During those times when my scale became impertinent and didn't report the expected results, those measurements helped me see progress. So did the photos. I wished I would have taken photos from multiple angles and more frequently. I could have added them to my journal.

Since so much has changed in my life and I am approaching three years of intermittent fasting, I revisit my original whys for intermittent fasting. This is what I know:

- I am healthy for my grandchildren
- I walk up even bigger hills without stopping or feeling short of breath
- I can easily look over both shoulders while driving and before I switch lanes
- I can put on pants without leaning against furniture
- I no longer have numbness in my hands or cramps in my feet
- My lipid profile has improved dramatically: my triglycerides are 64, and my HDL is 96
- I no longer have any guilt over my food choices
- I feel in control
- I no longer constantly crave sugar
- I am strong and mighty
- I tolerate summer heat
- I wear shorts (and bathing suits) in public

- My clothes are not too small from year to year, and I look better in them, but sometimes they are too big the next year (I didn't expect that problem)
- I don't mind having my picture taken
- Not only do I have a jawline; I have hipbones and visible collar bones
- I have muscle definition in my arms, legs, back, and shoulders
- I don't remember the last time I suffered from indigestion

As it turned out, my gums did improve according to my hygienist and periodontist. Autophagy took a while to reach my mouth, but now that it has, I am thrilled.

The fact that I no longer crave sugar is a biggie. I remember the days when each day without sugar was torture, and once I started eating, I wouldn't stop until it was gone or I was almost comatose from the sugar "high." Although I don't necessarily crave it, I occasionally partake. A single serving suits me, and I keep minimal amounts in the house. I no longer buy large quantities of cookies for the grandchildren and eat them all myself. I do keep ice cream in the freezer. I buy the best I can find—the full-fat and full-sugar versions. I indulge when I want and can go days without having any.

I continue the time-restricted eating version of intermittent fasting. I eat every day. I vary my fasting windows from 16 to 20 hours. I use an app to track my fasts—there are several free ones out there. I typically eat the same amount of food, regardless of the length of my fast, but there are days when I am just hungrier. So, I eat more. My goal is to keep my body guessing. I personally never fast longer than 24 hours. My body doesn't require it. Some people find that longer fasts (with mealless days) help their bodies heal and break through long plateaus. Others state that they have trouble sleeping after a mealless day. The beauty of intermittent fasting is that there are multiple ways to make it work and one size does not fit all!

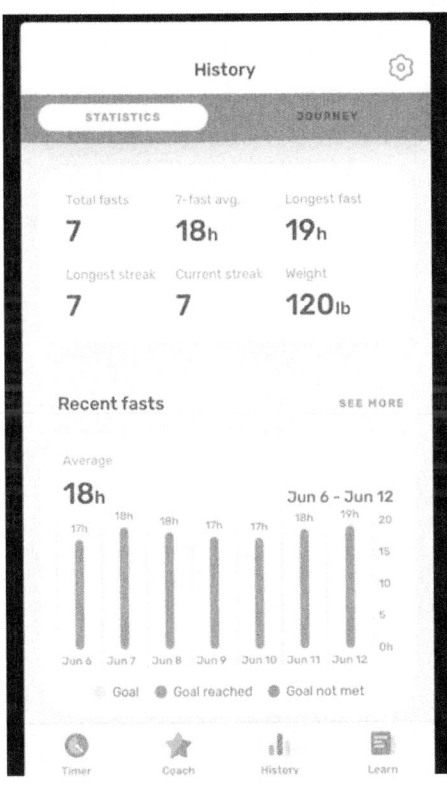

I miss my gym. I miss my pool. However, I have been consistent with my steps. I often get 150,000-plus steps/week and always over 100,000 each week. With shelter in place, I have a lot more time to walk. And I have begun running again—very slow speed but running. I know that I am running by the change in my gait—forefoot striking before my heel. Those that see me call it a walk because I am so slow. I feel that I burn more energy while running than walking, although the speeds are relatively equivalent. I run four to six miles a few times each week. And this running is different from my marathon training. It is an actual run. There is no more run/walk. I run the entire time.

I continue to plank and occasionally lift my seven-pound hand weights. I have no routine in this area, but I know the weights are important to my strength. I have discovered multiple activities that I enjoy. I water skied for the first time since my teens last summer at my brother's place. Yep, my arms felt like mush right after that, but I was able to get up and I wasn't sore the next day. I have surfed—although I confess, I only got up on my knees. I have paddle boarded, kayaked with the whales, and zip lined.

These days I talk about intermittent fasting to anyone who is curious, but I don't preach it. As a 64-year-old woman, do I wish I would have found intermittent fasting sooner? Yes and no. Part of me would have loved to avoid those sufferable diets, the weight gain that always occurred after the losses, those years of being overweight, the insults, and the self-shame. On the other hand, all of that makes me who I am today. I am a believer in intermittent fasting partially because of my previous failures. Winston Churchill once said, "Success is not final. Failure is not fatal. It is the courage that counts."

There is one person in our household who speaks of intermittent fasting more than I do—my husband. He proudly tells my story to neighbors, family members, and old friends. He doesn't always get the details of my eating window correct, but I forgive him because in every telling, he calls me "hot."

I have discovered my purpose: I babysit my grandchildren, as needed. I belong to a philanthropic group that provides financial resources for women's education. I am a moderator for Gin Stephen's Facebook Group: Delay, Don't Deny. I continue to attempt to be the best wife, mother, grandmother, sister, friend, and neighbor I can be.

Aside from being thinner and healthier, am I different from the person I was in early 2017? I am perhaps a little more confident and willing to take risks (thus, this book). I am also more content, grounded, and resilient. I am unsure if this is the result of intermittent fasting, retirement, or a combination of both. Either way, in this crazy time that we are living, I find value in these traits.

I sometimes wonder how I was able to maintain my weight loss this time, when I was unable to in the past. I think it is because this time I focused on the **process** of losing weight—intermittent fasting. In the past, I focused on the goal.

I was compelled to tell my story partially because so many others have experienced similar results. Some of them have lost over 200 pounds. I want everyone to have the knowledge and opportunity to conduct their own health experiment, get healthier, and find their thinner selves. For menopausal women, let my story give you hope.

I did not discover intermittent fasting. As it turns out, I was not one of the early adapters. However, I would like to share my health experiment since I spent an entire career as a health educator promoting methods that didn't work. If this book helps one person discover themselves with intermittent fasting, I will be thrilled.

I posted this photo in Delay, Don't Deny on 8/8/2020—my first size 0.

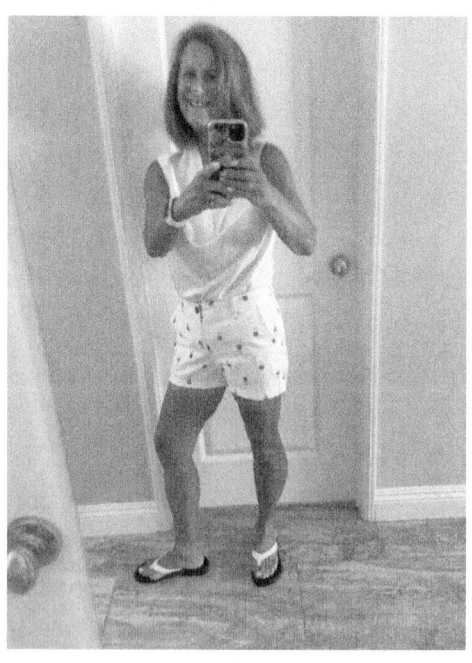

The comments to this selfie led me to believe that people wanted to hear my story. So perhaps my purpose is to tell it.

When we first locked down, I made one final in-person grocery-shopping run. We were told that we would have to rely on delivery indefinitely. There was very little on the shelves. The store was picked over of pastas, soups, cereals, and fresh and frozen fruits and vegetables. If I had been doing Weight Watchers or one of my many other diets, overall panic would have set in that I couldn't purchase my needed diet foods. Knowing we would have to eat something, I purchased what I could: meat, wine, chips, cheese, and crackers. I did not feel anxious. I could make a meal out of any of these things and continue intermittent fasting.

I have not had to make a New Year's resolution to lose weight since 2017. If you want to lose weight, keep it off, and get healthier in the process, I invite you to join me on the intermittent fasting journey.

PART TWO:
YOUR HEALTH EXPERIMENT

HOW TO GET STARTED

For some people, getting started is the hardest part. I get it. I was scared to start also. I was scared of failing...again. What if intermittent fasting doesn't work for me? What if I can't fast? First of all, everyone can fast because they do so when they fall asleep each night. It is just a matter of timing. And it will work for you, but sometimes it takes a while to see the results you are looking for.

Remember that you are designing and conducting an experiment to find health. You are the only participant. You need only commit to 30 days to start. You will be recording your daily observations in your journal.

When should you start? There is no better time like the present. Once you eat your dinner TODAY, start your first fast. If you aren't confident in your ability to fast 16 hours at the start, start where you know you can be successful. Set a goal that will guarantee your success and build confidence.

Consider how long you want to fast. Now consider how long you can promise to successfully fast. Start there. Is it 12 hours? 13 hours? Once you have completed a few shorter fasts, gradually extend by 15 minutes each day until you are at your desired fasting time. Remember that "Big doors swing on small hinges" (W.

Clement Stone). Start with the small actions to be performed consistently over time to produce giant changes in your life.

Of course, there are always people who don't believe in slow starts and want to be fasting 20 hours from day one. If you are confident in your ability to fast, jump in with both feet and choose a longer fast. Know you will be exchanging a challenging beginning with potentially faster results. If, by chance, you decide you need to change your approach, feel free to do so.

Once you have mastered the "true" fast—that is only drinking unflavored water, plain tea, and/or black coffee, you can consider extending your fasts a little longer. Be patient. The scale may not move at the beginning. Some bodies require significant healing, and that process begins once you start fasting.

I believe it helps to journal all of the reasons you want to lose weight. Some of those changes will happen sooner than others. Within the first month, I found it easier to look over my shoulder when switching lanes, but it took a year for me to feel totally comfortable in photos. Can you identify reasons that may happen sooner in your journey?

Take photos and measurements. Add them to your journal. There will be times that the scale is disrespectful and won't give you the feedback that you are looking for. The photos and measurements will be invaluable at that time.

A word about the scale: if your scale only gives you negative energy, don't weigh at all, or only once a month. If you can view the scale as a tool—the number on it as just a data point—then use the scale daily.

I cannot stress enough the value of journaling. Trends could go unnoticed if they aren't documented. Journaling led me to see which foods I couldn't control and, surprisingly, enjoy foods that I could. Remember how I said that I can't control my intake of jellybeans? You may wonder if all sugary foods set off a binge in me. Amazingly, I no longer appreciate most cakes and cookies enough to have more than one or two bites. I love ice cream but am satisfied with a small bowl. I learned all that from my journals.

I also find making a list of all things to be accomplished each day prior to eating has helped me maintain productivity and keep my fasting on track. When I worked full time out of the house, those lists were full of meetings, reports, discussions with co-workers, and rounds. As a retired person, I have had to become more creative. My lists today include my exercise plan for the day, errands to be run, tasks to be completed, people to call, and specific amounts to read in my current book. Your lists may look totally different.

People always ask: What happens if you are super-efficient and complete everything on your list prior to your fasting time being completed? I like to have another list of things that I would like to do someday, but it isn't urgent. This may include cleaning out an odd drawer, purging clothes as they become too big, and listening to an Intermittent Fasting Stories podcast by Gin Stephens (or other podcast) while I go for a walk. You can also listen to an audiobook. See below for more information on books and podcasts that I recommend.

If snacking after dinner is a problem for you, create a third list of things to do to avoid snacking. I found crocheting at night a great way to not nibble. Others enjoy a bath, or a long stroll with the dog. Be thoughtful and proactive. Having a friend to call at these times can be both therapeutic and relaxing. Some find a decaffeinated tea to sip while they reflect upon their day to be enjoyable. Board games or cards with your partner or roommate is another fun evening activity. Live alone? There are many computerized versions of games that can be played with others or versus the computer.

Through all of this—focus on the **process**—not the goal. Nail the process.

WORK ON YOUR BRAIN AS WELL AS YOUR BODY

Your brain has to get fit to maintain a healthy body. Forgive! Recognize that you may have had failed efforts at weight loss and forgive yourself. Remember that past results do not predict future outcomes. All past efforts have produced the wonderful you that is here today.

Be inspired! Have you ever heard the story of WD-40? WD-40 stands for "Water Displacement—40th attempt." In 1953, a small lab in San Diego set out to come up with a rust-prevention solvent and degreaser to be used in the aerospace industry. The first several attempts failed to achieve their desired results. In fact, their first 39 attempts failed. Did they give up? No! They got it right on the 40th attempt.

Believe! Believe that you can intermittently fast. Believe that intermittent fasting will work for you, but you will need to be patient. The weight won't disappear overnight. Consistency is the key. Until your body is metabolically able to burn both fat and glucose—usually two to four weeks into the journey—fasting will be hard. Keeping busy and mindful of your goals helps.

Hope! Jonas Salk once said, "Hope lives in dreams, in imagination, and in the courage of those who dare make dreams into reality." With hope you can fast. With hope you can become a new you!

View your time fasting as the magical time it is. Imagine your fat cells being released for energy during this time. Feel your body healing during your fast. Appreciate the mental clarity that is unmatched in a fasted state. Treasure the energy that fasting produces.

Consider intermittent fasting in ways that you can eat—not in ways you can't eat. Allow yourself to eat anything important to you within your window. Don't confuse eating anything with eating everything. Make choices that you are glad you made. Journal those choices, as well as the disappointments.

Recognize your body for its strengths—its ability to fast, move, carry you. Focus on those fabulous abilities. This is what your body does for you. Each day. Regardless of any previous abuse.

Watch the story your brain is telling. If you believe you can, you will. If you believe you can't, you won't. There are many studies that demonstrate this. If you continue to struggle with negative self-talk, implement the mantra: "Don't believe everything you think."

The biggest thought process to change is to think about where you want to be instead of where you are. This helps reframe those negative thoughts, as that negativity often inadvertently brings us exactly what we don't want.

TRUE FASTING AND FASTING LENGTH

What is true fasting? True fasting involves not imbibing in anything other than unflavored water (sparkling or still), plain, unflavored tea, and plain, unflavored coffee. Many will protest and argue in favor of cream in their coffee or artificial sweeteners during their fast. Let's explore why that is not recommended.

While adding cream, MCT oil, or butter may not take you out of ketosis, it will break your fast. An extremely limited self-study by Dr. Becky Gillaspy (a chiropractor) and her husband Keith showed that ingesting these fats with coffee maintained their ketosis (2018). That said, the calories in those foods break our fast. Our bodies return to burning ingested fats instead of the fat on our body for fuel. Our goal in intermittent fasting is to burn our body fat for fuel, so ingesting fats interrupts this goal.

Artificial sweeteners have served us well in our diet lives, so we believe(d). They provide sweetness without the added calories. Have they made us thin? Probably not, if you are reading this book. That said, many of us have enjoyed their added sweetness and may be unwilling to give them up. First of all, let's discuss them in your fast. Multiple studies have shown that ingesting sweet tasting things—even if there are no calories involved—spike insulin. And remember that those insulin spikes produce hunger. Even if you manage your fast, the insulin remains higher in our bodies, producing extreme hunger when you eat. We will discuss artificial sweeteners during our eating window later.

How long should a person fast is the million-dollar question. Fasting length depends upon your goals, your activity levels, what you eat within your window, your ability to fast, etc. People are unique in the length of fasts that work best for them at any given time. In fact, your own ideal fast length may, and probably will, change over time.

All that said, longer fasts may not produce greater weight loss than shorter fasts. In a recent study by the University of Illinois, both 20-hour fasts and 18-hour fasts produced comparable reductions of weight, insulin resistance, and oxidative stress over a 10-week period (Cienfuegos et al. 2020). Your study of one (YOU) will help you find your own perfect fasting length.

The goal is not to overeat in your window. If a shorter window causes you to overindulge, a longer window may serve you better. Be honest with yourself while trying to find your ideal window length. Also recognize your window length may change over time or from day to day.

Adam Sandler told Ellen DeGeneres that intermittent fasting made him so excited to eat within his window that he ate like it was a contest to eat as much as possible in his window. Understand this won't help you lose weight or get healthy. The amount of food consumed is a factor. It will make a difference in your success with intermittent fasting. Consider adding windowpanes to your eating window to help you limit your grazing. Remember that windowpanes are shorter time spans within your window where you will eat. So, if your eating window is six hours, you have specific times within that six hours where you rest and digest.

I was one of the lucky ones who was able to lose all of my weight primarily fasting 16 hours each day. Many require longer fasts to reach their goals. Others only get to goal by practicing alternate day fasting. I currently fast 16 – 20 hours each day to keep my body guessing and to hopefully improve autophagy.

BUT WHAT ABOUT HUNGER

The dictionary definition of "hunger" is discomfort accompanied by the desire to eat. Yep, following that definition led me to obesity. Accept the fact that you will feel hunger at the beginning. Also note that hunger comes in waves. When you hear your stomach growl, it is because your brain sent a message to your digestive tract to prepare for a meal. Both your brain and your digestive tract will forgive you if the meal does not come.

I remember being scared to death of hunger when I began my intermittent fasting journey. I felt hunger almost every minute of the day (Or at least I thought it was hunger. It may have just been food compulsion.). Once I began my fasting journey, I discovered hunger could roar but had a minimal bite. At first, seeing a time on the clock or available food made me ravenous. I instituted a "no free food" rule for myself. I didn't want to partake in food at work just because it was there. I rationalized that if I really wanted that particular food, I could purchase it myself and eat it in my window.

Note: Hunger is not unhealthy or an emergency. I know that contradicts what you have heard all your life. Consider your ancestors. They often missed meals. They often felt hunger. And then they ate food when it was available. It is important to note that our ancestors did not suffer from many of the chronic diseases that currently afflict modern society, such as type 2 diabetes, stroke, heart disease, and many cancers.

Words of advice: Don't be afraid of hunger and don't eat for future hunger. You may feel hunger at the same time each day. Welcome it like a good friend. Acknowledge its presence, and before you know it, the feeling of hunger will move on.

There are times in your fasting journey that you may be tempted to eat something now so you aren't hungry later. Make every effort to not fall into that trap. Chances are good that you may not even notice that wave of hunger later because you are being productive. If hunger does strike with a vengeance, that is when you can eat.

If, by chance, you get extreme physical symptoms of hunger, please eat. These symptoms may include, but are not necessarily limited to, shakiness, lightheadedness, and extreme weakness. As your body learns how to tap into its own fat stores, these symptoms will rarely occur.

THE EATING SIDE OF THE EQUATION

Many people struggle with the length of their eating window and foods to consume within that window. Let's start with the fact that the fast is the most important part. Nail the true fast! Got that part down? Now let's move on to the eating part.

Are you able to eat to satiety—eating until you are satisfied? Practice that. Eat less than you would normally eat and then wait. Are you satisfied? If not, adjust from there.

What to eat? What is the best diet? Well, isn't that the crucial quandary? Scientists have debated this notion for eons—well, maybe only centuries, but it seems like it forever. You can buy 10 books by 10 credible physicians and get 10 different and often conflicting opinions.

The truth on the best foods to support weight loss remains uncertain. For some it is high fat, while others do best with plant based. And others swear by nothing but animal-based products.

So, what is a person to eat? In a TED Talk by Eran Segal in 2016, he described how there is no one perfect diet for all humans. He explained how our DNA affects the way food works in our bodies. Researchers studied thousands of people who wore continuous glucose monitors and kept a food journal. Rice caused glucose spikes in some people but not others. Ice cream caused glucose spikes in some people but not others. As it turned out, all foods caused spikes in some people but not others. So, in other words, there are no "good" or "bad" foods. There are just foods that work better for each body.

A study published in 2019 (Berry et al.) takes this concept even further by looking at how both DNA and our own personal gut microbiome affected responses of the body to specific foods. They found out that the gut microbiome, our DNA, and the food itself contributed to how each body would respond to the specific food.

I believe we all have optimal diets. My perfect diet does not look like your perfect diet. I believe that most of us do best without significant amounts of highly processed foods. Aside from that, there are no rules that fit all of us.

How do you find which foods work best for you? By not eating continuously, you have a greater opportunity to pay attention to how your body responds to foods. Do some foods cause you to be hungrier after eating them? Do some foods cause you to retain fluids, become tired, or make you jittery? Journaling is your way of tracking those foods.

Amazingly, foods that affect you adversely now may no longer do so a few months from now. As our gut microbiomes become healthier, our bodies' reactions to foods can change. Although we have no ability to change our genes, we can positively impact our gut microbiome in just a couple of weeks. Tim Spector talks about how he can tell more about a person's health by way of a stool sample than a DNA sample.

Tim Spector also says that obesity is largely determined by our gut microbiome. A fatter person always has a less diverse microbiome than a thinner person. In fact, previously skinny people who have had fecal transplants (yes, that really is a thing for certain disease states) from an obese person, can find themselves rapidly gaining weight post-transplant.

In his book, The Diet Myth, Spector reported how 10 days of a McDonald's diet reduced microbiome diversity by 40 percent. In addition, artificial sweeteners can cause our guts to release toxins that can be detrimental to our gut microbiomes. There are YouTube videos where you can hear about Spector's work if you're curious.

A high-fiber diet is key to our gut health. Although fiber is known to be beneficial, what are the best sources? Multiple studies have shown that food fiber is far superior to supplemental fiber. So eat a variety of fruits and vegetables plus whole grains. Cheers to real food.

Many wonder how much food they should eat. If you were raised like me, your parents often asked you if you were full at the end of a meal. My four-year-old grandson will tell me he is too full to eat more chicken or carrots, but his tummy saved a space reserved for ice cream (yes, these are his words). Is there any question as to why we want to eat to fullness, when we should strive to eat to satiety—and yes, that includes the ice cream at times? There are better questions to ask ourselves. Before we eat, we should ask the following:

- Am I hungry?
- What do I want to eat?

- If I eat that now, will I still be happy with that decision an hour from now?

When we are new fasters, these answers won't be clear to us because we aren't used to listening to our bodies. As we become more experienced fasters, the answers become clearer and our choices change. Most people begin to choose fewer ultra-processed foods. Some choose more meat. Others choose more vegetables. What will your body choose?

Once you begin eating, you will want to pause and ask yourself the following: (ideally, you will recognize that point in a meal when you sigh. If not, practice putting your fork down mid meal)

- Am I still hungry?
- Am I satisfied? If I'm not satisfied, what do I want?

If you are uncertain of any of these answers, pause for 30 minutes and ask yourself again. The answers should be clearer.

HOW TO EMBRACE THE LIFESTYLE

A lifestyle is something you commit to do the rest of your life. Many diets sell themselves as lifestyles and, although I vowed I would continue them forever, within the first few weeks, I couldn't wait to quit. Each diet seemed to have something unsustainable for me. The worst part was the flexibility was limited.

I'm sure you've been on diets in the past where you reached a point where you "cheated." I know that this is my experience, and it isn't uncommon. Then I "fell off the wagon." Then I couldn't even find the wagon. With intermittent fasting there is no wagon. There are no "cheats." You only make choices. You decide what to eat and when to eat it. Are you craving ice cream? You decide when and how much to eat. Do you open your eating window earlier than you planned sometimes? Maybe. Will you occasionally eat after you have closed your window? Maybe. Will you love all your decisions? Probably not, especially those first few months, but that is alright.

We learn from those less-than-perfect decisions, especially if we are journaling. What are some of the things that you can expect to learn?

- Your ideal fasting length may vary over time

- Your body really will tell you the foods it needs and the amounts
- Intermittent fasting simplifies your life
- Intermittent fasting can improve your focus and productivity

So dump the wagon mentality. It will not help you. Embrace the flexibility of intermittent fasting.

WHAT YOU CAN EXPECT TO GET WITH AN INTERMITTENT FASTING LIFESTYLE

I began intermittent fasting to lose weight, as do many others. The good news is that intermittent fasting has multiple health benefits. Autophagy is one. Autophagy is magic that can happen in our bodies to recycle broken down pieces at a cellular level. It is important to note that exercise is also a big promoter of autophagy. So, although exercise does not always produce weight loss, its benefits cannot be overlooked due to its promotion of autophagy.

The exploration into the benefits of autophagy remains incomplete but impressive. We know it promotes longevity, protects against many chronic diseases, such as cancer and fatty liver disease, and may be our best defense against Alzheimer's.

Autophagy slows down the aging process by cleaning house at the cellular level. Our cells are constantly being damaged by our acts of living: digestion, immunity, energy conversion, etc. With age and stress and exposure to certain environmental toxins, our cells face even greater damage. If these damaged cells remain, our bodies react with inflammation and specific disease processes. Autophagy is our bodies' house cleaning and recycling of these damaged cells.

Autophagy has shown to produce multiple benefits:

- Helps cells to burn fuel efficiently and make proteins from recycled cellular material, thus increasing metabolism
- Reduces risks of neurogenerative diseases
- Helps regulate inflammation
- Helps fight infectious diseases
- Improves muscle performance
- Prevents cancer onset
- Improves digestive health
- Improves skin health

Intermittent fasting can reduce oxidative stress and inflammation in the body, thus decreasing the chances of many chronic diseases. It also improves many markers for heart disease, including blood pressure, total and LDL cholesterol, triglycerides, and blood sugar. Fasting has been shown to have several effects on metabolism that may reduce the risk for many types of cancers. In addition, fasting has been shown to be beneficial for brain health and actually prevent Alzheimer's.

Since I am hoping for increased autophagy and other health benefits, I aim for longer fasts although I am in maintenance.

BOOKS AND PODCASTS

Although I started intermittent fasting without reading a single book, I reached a point when I wanted to learn more and began reading books, then listening to podcasts. Here are some of my favorites:

BOOKS:

Delay, Don't Deny by Gin Stephens: This book is written in conversational style and includes all the information on how intermittent fasting works scientifically (without too much scientific jargon) and everything you need to know to get started. This is the book that showed me that fasting clean makes a difference.

Feast, Fast, Repeat, also by Gin Stephens, is a book written in her conversational style but includes many more studies. This book also sheds some light on the eating window side of the equation.

The Obesity Code by Jason Fung provides all the background science of intermittent fasting. He also wrote The Diabetes Code, beneficial for those with Type 2 Diabetes.

The Diet Myth by Tim Spector is a fabulous book about why specific foods work for one person but not another. He digs deep into his studies of both genetics and the gut microbiome.

PODCASTS:

The Intermittent Fasting Stories: These are interviews between Gin Stephens and people who are Intermittent Fasting and are very inspirational. Listen to all of these.

Intermittent Fasting Podcast by Melanie Avalon and Gin Stephens: a podcast to burn fat, gain energy, and enhance wellness.

The Peter Attia Drive Podcast: an expert insight into health, performance, and longevity with an intermittent fasting spin.

BODY RECOMPOSITION

I remember my first few months of intermittent fasting, where my weight decreased significantly, but I couldn't fit into smaller clothes yet. Last summer I was definitely a size 6 on the bottom and a 10 on top—due to the continued presence of my boobs. I purchased my entire—hopefully for life—wardrobe. This summer, the dresses still look great, but the size 6 shorts, pants, etc., are way too big.

Have I lost additional weight? Maybe two to three pounds. Is it my imagination? Not at all. My body has changed. Many others have reported dramatic changes in their bodies without changing their weight with intermittent fasting. If you do not believe me, look online for pictures. That is why we recommend taking pictures.

Why does this happen? First, you are burning fat and maintaining muscle. Also there is clear evidence that human growth hormone is increased while fasting, stimulating more muscle growth and bone density. Also, your loose skin may shrink (which is related to increased autophagy). These changes can produce amazing changes in photos and measurements without a scale change.

It is important to realize that your body may continue to change well after weight loss stops with continued intermittent fasting. So accept this as a known side effect, even if it means you will need to buy smaller sizes.

SUPPLEMENTS AND VITAMINS

Many people will ask which vitamins and supplements I used on my intermittent fasting journey. Here is my full disclosure: I used no vitamins or supplements during that first year. I now occasionally take magnesium gluconate to help with sleep. I consulted with my physician, who has approved the supplement for this use. I recommend consulting with your physician prior to using any supplements. None are required for intermittent fasting.

As a side note, there are multiple products on the market that measure your ketones, your blood sugar, and the foods that you are burning for energy. I used none of those. I relied on how my body felt and the objective numbers that we all have readily available—weight, measurements, etc.

SUPPORT FROM THE EXPERTS

It has taken a while for physicians to jump on board the intermittent fasting band wagon. You can't blame them. They had been taught about calories in versus calories out and the food pyramid. Many smart people—not just Jason Fung—have been praising the value of intermittent fasting.

Mark Mattson, Ph.D. began exploring intermittent fasting as a way to slow the aging process in the early 2000s. He promoted the 5:2 method as a way to lose weight and improve health. He declared that fasting preserved brain health in his 2014 TED Talk (and probably earlier to others.). He referenced a book written over 100 years ago by Upton Sinclair called The Fasting Cure. (The entire book can be found online.) He interviewed 250 people and determined that fasting had improved or eliminated their symptoms. He went on the speak about the benefits of fasting to the body:

- Decreased insulin
- Increased ketones
- Increased insulin sensitivity
- Reduced inflammation
- Improved cognitive function
- Increased stress resistance
- Reduced resting heart rate

- Reduced blood pressure
- Lipolysis—the breakdown of fats

Michael Mosley, a British physician and television journalist, popularized the 5:2 plan with his BBC broadcast, "Eat Fast, Live Longer in 2012." This was followed by his book, The Fast Diet. Mosley had put himself on the plan to lose weight and reverse his newly diagnosed type 2 diabetes.

Dr. Bert Herring also used intermittent fasting to treat himself. He was one of the first to subscribe to a time-restricted eating plan. Both he and his wife fell into a 19:5 plan that worked for both of them. His 2013 TED Talk spoke of a plan for water skiing at 100 years of age as a benefit of intermittent fasting. He talked about the industrial influence to just eat! Eat—make everyone happy! However, he recognized how much better he felt when he didn't eat; when he skipped meals.

Mark Mattson and Rafael de Cabo, Ph.D. coauthored an article in the New England Journal of Medicine supporting the benefits of intermittent fasting. This article promoted the benefits of intermittent fasting to improve health, increase longevity, and decrease disease processes. If your physician has not heard about intermittent fasting, call out this article from 12/26/19.

Peter Attia is a physician who focuses on longevity. He believes that intermittent fasting increases longevity but promotes the need for dosage—how much fasting is required to produce the desired results.

THE HEALTH EXPERIMENT

Rob Jones of the Utah Wellness Institute uses intermittent fasting as one way to balance hormones. He has treated over 500 patients with intermittent fasting, in conjunction with other treatments. He discovered intermittent fasting from a couple of patients in 2014 before he began using it has a treatment.

Other physicians, such as Dr. Clark-Ganheart, lost weight and healed themselves before promoting intermittent fasting to their patients. She began with longer fasts but settled into an 18:6 pattern that works for her. She no longer needs the antihypertensive medication she was taking previously.

MANAGE YOUR STRESS

Chronic stress can have a dramatic response on our bodies by producing cortisol and causing unhealthy stress-related behaviors, resulting in weight gain. When you are stressed, your adrenal glands produce adrenaline and cortisol. The adrenaline sends glucose into your bloodstream to provide the needed energy to "fight or flight"—get out of that dangerous situation. Once the threat is no longer apparent, this glucose high plummets, resulting in cravings for sugar. The cortisol that is released is an appetite stimulant and metabolism reducer. In the "fight or flight" situation, cortisol temporarily pauses normal bodily functions, thus slowing the metabolism.

A 2014 study by Ohio State University (Kiecolt-Glaser et al.) showed that women who had experienced a stressful event in the previous 24 hours burned over 100 fewer calories than non-stressed women. So, not only does anxiety not burn extra calories; it actually conserves them. Our bodies metabolize slower under stress. This same study showed that stressed women had higher levels of insulin in their bodies than non-stressed women. Remember that insulin causes us to store fat. Stress also causes unhealthy behaviors, such as emotional eating and sleep deprivation.

I know we can't predict or prevent all stressors, but we can manage our responses to them. The following are ways to manage the stress:

- Exercise
- Meditation
- Healthy eating
- Enjoy nature
- Call a friend
- Take a bubble bath
- Get a massage
- Read a book
- Listen to music
- Deep breathing
- Most importantly, make self-care a priority

SAVE TIME AND MONEY

Preparing less frequent meals means you will save time. I remember packing meals and snacks in previous "diets" to take to work. I had containers of all sizes because everything had to be weighed and measured prior to consuming. I could spend over a half hour prepping my food bag for work, then need to spend time after work washing all the containers. Also, remember the time and mental energy required to track everything you ate? I recall reviewing menus prior to eating out to determine what would fit best into my plan. None of that is required for intermittent fasting.

Have you noticed that in no place in this book is there a requirement or recommendation for you to buy into a program or purchase special foods or supplements? Intermittent fasting requires no financial commitment. Let me repeat that. Intermittent fasting requires no financial commitment! In fact, you may find that your grocery bill is reduced. Save that money for new clothes because you are going to need them.

CONCLUSION

Ralph Waldo Emerson said, "All life is an experiment. The more experiments you make the better." Don't miss this opportunity to find a healthier and happier self. And say goodbye to weight loss as a New Year's resolution!

REFERENCES

Berry, Sarah, Ana Valdes, Richard Davies, Linda Delahanty, David Drew, Andrew Chan, Nicola Segota, Paul Franks, and Tim Spector. "Predicting Personal Metabolic Responses to Food using Multi-Omics Machine Learning in Over 1000 Twins and Singletons from the UK and US: The Predict I Study." In *Current Developments in Nutrition*, no. 3 (June 2019).

Cienfuegos, Sofia, Kelsey Gabel, Faiza Kalam, Shihou Lin, Manoela Oliveira, and Krista Varady. "Effects of 4- and 6-h Time-Restrictive Feeding on Weight and Cardiometabolic Health: A Randomized Controlled Trial on Adults with Obesity." In *Cell Metabolism*, no. 32 (July 15, 2020): 366-378.

Cox, Carla. "Role of Physical Activity for Weight Loss and Weight Maintenance." In *Diabetes Spectrum*, no. 30 (Aug 2017): 157-160.

Crum, Alia, William Corbin, Kelley Brownell, and Peter Salovey. "Mind Over Milkshakes: Mindsets, Not Just Nutrients Determine Ghrelin Response." In *Health Psychology*, no. 30 (July 2011): 430-431.

Dehghan, Mashhad, Andrew Mente, Xiaohe Zheng, Samanthi Swaminathan, Wei Li, Viswanathan Mohan. "Associations of Fat and Carbohydrate Intake with Cardiovascular Disease and Mortality in 18 Countries from Five Continents (PURE): A Prospective Cohort Study." In *The Lancet*, no. 390 (August 29, 2017): 2050-2062.

Dr. Becky Fitness, "Coffee Experiment! What Can I Put in My Coffee When Intermittent Fasting—We Ran the Test." Accessed August 8, 2020. https://drbeckyfitness.com/coffee-and-intermittent-fasting.

Hall, Kevin and Scott Kahan. "Maintenance of Lost Weight and Long Term Management of Obesity." In *The Medical Clinics of North America*, no. 102 (Jan 2018): 183-197.

Howell, Scott and Richard Kones. "'Calories In, Calories Out' and Macronutrient Intake: The Hope, Hype, and Science of Calories." In the *American Journal of Physiology— Endocrinology and Metabolism*, no. 313 (Nov. 29, 2017): 608-612.

Kiecolt-Glaser, Janice, Diane Habash, Christopher Fagundes, Rebecca Andridge, Juan Peng, William Malarkey, and Martha Balury. "Daily Stressors, Past Depression, and Metabolic Responses to High Fat Meals: A Novel Path to Obesity." In *Biological Psychiatry*, no. 77 (July 2014): 653-660.

Lee, I-Min, Eric Shiroma, and Matsamisu Kamada. "Association of Step Volume and Intensity with All Cause Mortality in Older Women." In the *Journal of American Medical Association*, no. 179 (May 29, 2019): 1105-1112.

Mathur, Kushagra, Kumar Rashat, Shailesh Nagpure, and Depalli Deshpande. "Effect of Artificial Sweeteners on

Insulin Resistance among Type-2 Diabetes Mellitus Patients." In *Journal of Family Medicine and Primary Care*, no. 9 (Jan 2020): 69-71.

Mazzotti, Diego, Camila Guindalini, and Sergio Tufik. "Human Longevity is Associated with Regular Sleep Patterns, Maintenance of Slow Wave Sleep, and Favorable Lipid Profile." In *Front Paging Neuroscience*, no. 6 (2014): 134.

Popkin, Barry, Shufa Du, William Green, Melinda Beck, Taghred Algaith, Christopher Herbst, Reem Alsukait, Mohammed Alluhidan, Nahar Alazemi, and Meera Shekar. "Individuals with Obesity and Covid-19: A Gloval Perspective on Epidemiology and Biological Relationships." In *Obesity Reviews*, no. 21 (August 2020).

Saint-Maurice, Pedro, Richard Troiano, and David Basset. "Association of Daily Step Count and Step Intensity with Mortality among US Adults." In the *Journal of American Medical Association*, no. 323 (March 24/31, 2020): 1151-1160.

Yang, Yi-Long, Li Liu, Xiang-Xi Wang, Yang Wang, and Lie Wang. "Prevelance and Associated Positive Psychological Variables of Depression and Anxiety among Chinese Cervical Cancer Patients." In the *Public Library of Science*, no. 9 (2014).

Printed in Great Britain
by Amazon